EVERY WOMAN'S HERBAL

by
Dr. John R. Christopher, N.D., M.H.

with
Cathy Gileadi

D1421727

ISBN 1-879436-10-8

This edition published in August 1994
by Christopher Publications
P.O. Box 412
Springville, UT 84663

Printed in the United States of America

SPECIAL NOTE TO THE READER

This edition of *Every Woman's Herbal* includes a new section on cleansing during pregnancy and added information on immunizations. We have revised dated information to show current status and replaced a complex pad pattern with a more effective, simple one. Also included is review work on new products that have appeared on the market since the last printing, new recipes, art work, and additional case histories. Other minor revisions and textual corrections plus a more extensive index provide a more pleasant and informative reading.

-The editors, staff and Cathy Gileadi

EVERY WOMAN'S HERBAL
TABLE OF CONTENTS

PREFACE

INTRODUCTION I

PUBERTY 1

BEFORE CHILDBEARING 12

PREGNANCY.. 25
  Morning sickness, Weight Gain, Technology, Exercise,
  Constipation, Anemia, Indigestion, Backache, Muscle
  Pain, Varicosities, Urinary Infections, Yeast Infections,
  Toxemia, High Blood Pressure, Hormones, Miscarriage,
  Vitamins, Rh Factor, Vaginal Birth After Caesarean.

BIRTH 50
  High Risk for Home Birth, Midwifery and Law, Onset of
  Labor, Preparatory Labor, Self Exam, Prenatal Formula,
  Supplies for Home Birth, Baby Clothes, Labor Herbs,
  Reflexology and Birth, Energy Giving Herbs, Pain,
  Expelling the Placenta, Hemorrhage, Shock, Perineal
  Hygiene, After Pains, Engorgement, Breast Infection.

THE NEW BABY 85
  Silver Nitrate, Conjunctivitis, Formula, Early Nursing,
  Exclusive Breastfeeding , Nursing, Weaning, Serious
  Illness, Yeast Infection in Babies, Jaundice, Constant
  Contact, Circumcision, Colic, Diaper Rash, Dry Skin,
  Cradle Cap, Colds and Fevers, Fever, Teething,
  Vomiting, Diarrhea, Ear Infection, Immunizations.

Continued...

TABLE OF CONTENTS

Continuation

HEALTHY WOMAN..109
    Reproductive System, Incurables, Cancer, Bone Cancer,
    Breast Cancer, Multiple Sclerosis, Influenza,
    Gallstones, Cysts and Tumors, Gas, Asthma, Drug
    Abuse, Vision Troubles, Gangrene,
    Diabetes/Hypoglycemia, Hair Loss, Deafness/Ear
    Troubles, Pyorrhea, Constipation, Overweight,
    Osteoporosis, Reflexology, Headaches, Emotional
    Health, Insomnia, PMS, Yeast Infection, Technology,
    Urinary Infection, Heart Disease, Allergies.

FIRST AID...158

MENOPAUSE...168

THE THREE-DAY CLEANSE, HERBAL CLEANSE,
MUCUSLESS DIET. & HERBAL FORMULAS....................171
    Three-Day Cleanse, Herbal Cleanse, Mucusless Diet,
    Recipes, Herbal Formulas

PREPARATIONS...204

REFERENCES..211

INDEX 214

PREFACE

What a find! What a wonderful treasure! Three years after Dr. Christopher's death, we find a 100 page manuscript on women, filed and forgotten. We employed the aid of his good friend, Cathy Gileadi, who is an excellent writer, and we present to you this beautiful herbal for women.

Unlike other herbals that list this herb for this complaint and that herb for that complaint, this work explains and details the root of the problems. Dr. Christopher then outlines a wholistic approach for overcoming the malady.

Every Woman's Herbal is like a novel that you won't want to put down. We recommend that you read the book in its entirety, and then use the excellent index as a reference guide.

Dr. Christopher was a true teacher, in every sense of the word, and those who knew him personally know that he would teach in a way that would not offend or hurt. However, his stand against abortion is meant as a warning, not as a condemnation for those unfortunate enough to have been subjected to the surgeon's ignorance or defiance to human life.

We release this book with hopes of touching the lives of many.

David W. Christopher
Christopher Publications

INTRODUCTION

While he was still with us, Dr. Christopher had been compiling experiences and stories for a woman's herbal. We are pleased to present his work and to add information from current research on natural healing for women.

Dr. Christopher's empathy for women began early in life. As an orphan, abandoned by his parents when only a newborn, he felt a keen sense of love for his adopted family, and a great desire to feel part of an intact family. His adopted mother suffered from diabetes and arthritis, for which Raymond treated her with standard remedies throughout his young years. Later the diabetes developed into Bright's Disease, Bright's Disease into dropsy (edema); then gangrene set in and she swelled to many times her normal size. Her intense suffering--and the medical profession's inability to relieve it--started Dr. Christopher on the road which led to the principles of diet and health that he taught. In his own words, "I was filled with a sense of burning pity and helpless rage at the unfairness of it all. I was naive enough to believe that God rewards people as good as my mother with good, certainly not with so many years of pain and suffering, followed by a painful, agonizing death. I recalled our Church's Word of Wisdom, which promised health to those who would keep that law. My mother kept this Word of Wisdom, as we then understood it; she did not use tea, coffee, liquor or tobacco! Why then did God break His promise, I asked myself? After many years of studying and rereading this scripture, I found that the 'diet' part had been ignored. I watched my mother die, and I vowed that someday I would be able to help people, to keep them from this type of suffering."

Throughout his practice, Dr. Christopher made it a point to help women attain their true feminine potential. During a time of rampant abortion, he insisted that women were meant to bear children and raise families. He would often cite, with strong emotion, the good that parents can do in raising healthy, moral children. When unhappy prospective mothers came to him seeking an herbal abortifacient, he discouraged them. For example, when he was practicing in Salt Lake City, the receptionist called, saying that a lady had come in without an appointment. Dr. Christopher only had a few moments until his next appointment was due to arrive, but this young woman claimed that she wanted no eye readings nor adjustments, but just a few moments to talk. Dr. Christopher agreed to see her, and she entered, a belligerent young lady. He asked her to take a seat, which she refused. She said, "I want to get rid of this brat that's in me. Give me something to get rid of it. I don't want it!"

Though he had only a few minutes to spare, Dr. Christopher sat her down and made her listen. He spoke to her for about forty-five minutes, telling her that getting rid of her fetus would be murder, one of the crudest things she could do. He advised her to let it come to earth, and to take care of it. Throughout his advice, she would interrupt rebelliously. After forty-five minutes of this, she stood up, glared at him, and declared, "If I had a gun, I'd kill you! I just hate you! And I'm going to get rid of this thing in me by some other doctor."

Dr. Christopher assured her that she could choose whatever she wished, but she should remember all the things he had told her. Time passed, and he forgot all about this young lady's visit. A year later, however, the receptionist announced a young lady who wanted to speak to Dr. Christopher for just a moment. It was the same young woman who had responded with venom to his counsel. She walked in, a changed person, carrying in her arms one of the sweetest little babies the Doctor had ever seen. She said she wanted to thank him. "This baby has changed my life," she said, "It's the most beautiful thing I could have ever received. Once I wanted to kill you, but I am glad you told me what you did. I went to two or three other doctors, who put me on their waiting list for abortions, but each time I would go to see them, I would remember what you had told me, and I'd get up and walk out before they'd ever see me. I carried the baby full-term--and here it is!"

Although Dr. Christopher stressed the importance of women having children (he often said that it was a shame that so many women were aborting children, while there were so many others who were anxious and sorrowful because they could not conceive), he did not minimize the important contributions that women make outside of the family. When he was writing his books, I helped him by doing research, editing and writing for him. Being right in the middle of my childbearing years, I could not leave my home to compete in the business world, yet Dr. Christopher still employed me. In the production of his Childhood Diseases (now called *Herbal Home Health Care*) he would drive thirty-five miles from his home to mine to deliver parts of the manuscript. When I would phone to tell him the work was complete, he would drive the same distance to pick it up, always paying me fairly and always praising me for what I did. (What consideration for a young mother working out of her own home, and what an opportunity!) He could have hired someone more easily available out in the work force, but he chose to give a woman the opportunity to work and to stay at home with her children.

Perhaps in reaction to the pressures of radical feminism, more and more women--and men--of all ages are leaving the pressures of the work world to create a preferable environment at home. For a woman, staying home demands discipline rarely achieved in the workplace. If she runs a home business, she must integrate it into the needs of the household--an organizational feat, one that stretches her capacities and leads her along the path of spiritual growth. If she does not earn at home, she has time to learn skills or study subjects that she might otherwise have missed. "Why go to college?" a young woman once asked me, "I can learn anything I want by studying from books." (And, incidentally, colleges around the world are granting credit for such study; some of them consider it superior to what is force-learned in classrooms.) Many professionals of both sexes consider the pressures of working in large companies, or of doing work they don't really enjoy, not worth the price. They give up the higher pay or better benefits for more control of their lives. Healthwise, the important thing is to find peace, to feel in control of one's life, to have balance between what must be done to earn a living and what we want to do to nurture our families, to expand our minds, and to refine ourselves generally. Without that balance, we can enter dis-ease. By being truly happy in our day-to-day activities, we can build our health as well.

Robert A. Johnson, in a fascinating book exploring the Eros/Psyche myth, suggests that "every woman needs to learn to relate with courage to the outer world, but she knows instinctively that too much of it at once is fatal, and even to go near it is dangerous. Imagine a very feminine woman at the beginning of her lifework, looking at the modern world and knowing that she must make her way through it...One can be bludgeoned to death, depersonalized by the ram nature of the patriarchal, competitive, impersonal society in which we live." (Johnson, *She*, San Francisco: Harper & Row, p. 50.)

By far the most significant time to stay home is a woman's childbearing years. Editors John and Peggy McMahon of *Mothering Magazine* think it is ideal for *both* parents to work at home when children are young. They can then both participate in the difficulties and delights of childbearing together, and the children benefit from both role models. Instinctively we sense that the best parenting a child can receive comes from his natural parents -with babies, especially the mother. Something is born in a woman when her child enters the world; she is gifted with a special insight, knowing what her child needs. One breastfeeding specialist recognized this, telling mothers to watch their babies for the messages which will tell them exactly what to do; she equates the always-accurate inner voice to the Holy Spirit. An energy akin to nourishment passes from parent to child--and back again in a never-ending cycle. A caretaker can never duplicate that.

Not only the childbearing years bear fruit for a stay-at-home woman, however. Many middle-aged and older women find peace and growth in gardening, study, crafts (in the elegant sense, such as basketmaking and weaving), writing, and, of course, herb collecting and processing. From my experience, the superiority of an eight-to-five rat race is a mere delusion. And women in Russia, who have all been liberated and, therefore, are all permitted to hold jobs, feel the same. Hedrick Smith, describing Russian life, devotes an entire chapter to the condition of women. "Away with your emancipation!" one responded when questioned about women's liberation. "After the Revolution when they emancipated women, it meant that women could do the same heavy work as men. But many women prefer not to work but to stay at home and raise their children. I have one child but I wanted more but who can afford more children? Unfortunately, we cannot *not work* because the pay our husbands earn is not enough to live on. So we have to go every day and make money" (Hedrick Smith, *The Russians*, New York: Ballantine, 1976, page 177).

Many Americans are not as financially strapped as the Russians are--although the economic pressure seems to be on more than ever--but many women feel obligated to do "something" with their lives instead of living them fully at home.

Not everyone need stay at home, of course. In some families, the woman prefers to work out of the home while the man takes care of the children. The bottom line is to find the thing that makes us happy, content, balanced. Most of us know women who are thoroughly absorbed in their work, thoroughly happy. But we must not be taken in by claims that all women would be happier working away from home. My mother, for example, assured us that she was delighted with her highly-placed executive post in state government, complete with large office and staff. However, all at once she decided it was too stressful and didn't really satisfy her; she gave it all up to offer a home for disturbed women. This keeps her interested and occupied, and she is offering something of herself to those who need her.

With whatever time we have for quiet nurture, we can remember that Dr. Christopher always taught that the best healing plants and foods come from our own back yards. To till the soil, plant the seeds, put in fruit trees, and let the medicinal "weeds" thrive in our own yards, picking them at just the right time for each, enjoying the sun and wind and rain--this kind of life cannot be compared with any financial benefits from the sterile treadmill that the business world can sometimes be. Our homes and families should provide us the peace and balance that can help us maintain perfect health.

So this herbal is somewhat different from others you may have used. Instead of giving you a list of possible herbs to use in order to heal yourself, we take the point of view that healing results from at least three approaches: nutrition, exercise, and mental balance. Without each of these, you can attain only a certain measure of health. Some of our friends eat a really good diet, but their life situation subjects them to tremendous stress, and they only get intermittent exercise. They are ill sometimes, and don't feel good, because they are only experiencing one-third of the healing program.

Dr. Christopher often emphasized the healing aspects of the natural environment. He encouraged people to walk barefoot on the grass or sand to help discharge pent-up energies and tensions. He suggested a daily sunbath, even in the wintertime by using a tent constructed on a clothesline to trap warmth. He taught deep breathing, to take in the breath of life, and we hope that breath draws in unpolluted air.

Dr. Christopher shared the ingredients of his formulas freely, for he was often given the combinations from God. He usually recommended simple herbs, the common ones that grow wild around us. Following his example, we suggest only a few herbs or combinations for various ailments or conditions. These herbs work. But we suggest at the end of a section other alternatives, in case you cannot obtain the ones we best recommend.

Don't accept the common notion that only a skilled pharmacist can understand the workings of herbs enough to safely use them. Used correctly, none of the herbs we suggest here can harm you. Use them with wisdom and prudence, and you will learn their various properties as you go along.

The chapter on herbal "Preparations," page 204, will guide you in making the preparations. You will be surprised how easy it is to make up the various herbs. When you make your first herbal tincture or oil, you'll feel tremendous satisfaction and enjoyment.

Remember that herbs usually work slowly, when a person is in fair health. It may take months or even a year or two to overcome a chronic condition. We always say that it may take as long to get over a problem as it took to develop it, although this is not always the case. When a person is in a crisis, often the herb will effect a marvelous and dramatic cure.

Herbs cleanse and cure, and sometimes their workings will mystify us. For example, a woman was working on an herbal thesis, deciding to write about the herb bladderwrack. She decided to experiment with bladderwrack to have some personal experience with the herb. Every time she took it, she got a severe bladder infection. She tried increasing the dose, but the infection just got worse. When she stopped taking the herb, the infection stopped. Needless to say, she was mystified.

Analyzing the situation, she decided that this area of her body must need cleansing. Before she had started on a natural diet and program, she had treated bladder infections with standard medical procedure, that is, antibiotics. Perhaps she was experiencing a weakness in her system. So she continued taking the bladderwrack and suffering with the infections. Soon they cleared completely and she never had any more trouble with the area.

David Christopher, Dr. Christopher's herbalist son, suggested that she would have gotten over the problem even faster if she had taken blood-cleansing herbs, hot baths, and the three-day cleanse. When we see that an herb is having a dramatic cleansing effect on us, we can feel thankful and use the other cleansing methods to speed the healing.
In all my personal experiences with herbs, I have never been disappointed. We even treat our animals herbally, and our children ask for chamomile tea for headache, or comfrey ointment for a scrape.

I hope that this Woman's Herbal can bring a degree of health (and self-sufficiency) that you may never have experienced before.

PUBERTY

Too many of us recall with distaste the time we became women. Instead of rejoicing as we crossed the threshold from childhood to young womanhood, we suffered shame, embarrassment, and pain from menstrual cramps. Perhaps we were uninformed and terrified at the flow; one young woman confided that she was certain that she was dying when her first period commenced, for her mother had never explained puberty to her. Most often, our mothers' hasty and uncomfortable explanations colored our emotional reactions to menstruation.

How lovely it is for a girl to become a woman! Her body shape changes and she begins the path to motherhood when she first menstruates. Some Native American tribes celebrate with the whole community when a girl reaches womanhood, with special ceremonies, dances, and gifts. Many modern mothers, having overcome their negative feelings about menstruation, are helping their young daughters celebrate their "rite of passage" into womanhood. Sometimes the mother fashions a special menstrual pad out of satin or silk, trimming it with embroidery or ribbon. After the pad is used, mother and daughter ceremonially bury it as a symbol of childhood now past. Some girls wear a pretty skirt, a special ribbon, or other adornment at the time of their periods, signifying a heightened and joyful attitude toward their bodies' cycle. Mothers help their daughters understand the emotional and energy changes related to their cycles, using these changes to plan their monthly activities; they are most active during the time after menstruation, when their energies are concentrated, and then as the period approaches, the girl learns to be more meditative and quiet. How wonderful to have a mother guide a young woman through these changes!

Too often, however, young people's systems are so out of balance that puberty becomes nightmarish for them. They suffer from acne oily skin, large pores, sometimes all over the face, chest and back. They become touchy, irritable, snappish; sometimes they are depressed, sometimes ecstatic. Why all these changes?

It takes a lot of energy and building materials to change from a girl to a woman. When she fills her body with low-energy, devitalized junk food, a girl cannot obtain the vital nutrition she needs to grow. Her body may be crying out for the natural hormone and estrogen materials it needs; it may be starving for the vitamins, minerals and enzymes it lacks. With so many junk foods at hand, most young people stuff themselves, and yet feel hungry. We can call this "hidden hunger," resulting because the foods eaten have not supplied our needs. Often the girl's menstrual cycle can be early or late, with cramps and systemic misery.

What can we do about these extremes? Dr. Christopher recommended the mucusless diet, with plenty of fruits, vegetables, grains, nuts and seeds. He observed families who raised their children on these foods from the time they were small. As teenagers, the children suffered no acne and no anger; they went through puberty with their sweet dispositions still intact!

A girl approaching puberty should drink a cup (or more) of red raspberry leaf tea daily and the same of blessed thistle tea. These supply the estrogen materials her body will require. Continue to drink these throughout the teenage years. They taste pleasant, and you can sweeten them and cool them in the refrigerator for a healthy substitute for soft drinks.

Some girls crave licorice root, which is a hormonal herb. It makes a good-tasting tea, hardly requiring any honey to sweeten, also very nice cold. We like to buy the licorice roots and chew on them, which also relieves nervous tension. Sarsaparilla is an excellent hormonal herb; make up a strong tea, sweeten and chill it, and add a bit of sparkling mineral water for a really nice treat.

If you happen to suffer from menstrual cramps, try some of the following. Catnip tea is a great pain reliever and general relaxant. Take it sweetened with honey, nice and hot. It can also bring on delayed menstruation. Another favorite for these uses is chamomile tea. Sometimes, if you have enough chamomile around for this purpose, you can make a very strong brew and add it to a hot bath for pain relief and relaxation. Basil, marjoram, and thyme--the common kitchen friends--make up into relaxing and pain-relieving teas. Hot ginger tea can bring on a delayed period and relieve cramps.

Other herbs used for painful menstruation, which is also called dysmenorrhea, are black cohosh, chaparral, cramp bark, squaw vine, true unicorn, valerian, and wild yam. You can also try taking more red raspberry leaf tea than usual to relieve the pain.

Try hot baths with the addition of any of these teas. Sometimes a walk in the sun and fresh air will cleanse the body of toxins which aggravate the condition, although you may have to talk yourself into going. Chiropractic adjustments may relieve pressures in the area that cause real menstrual pain. One teenage girl we know enjoyed her first painless period at age eighteen. A naturopath/chiropractor worked on her back and zones in her body, relieving enough pressure that the period came easily.

If you, like other young women, dislike purchasing expensive and sometimes irritating menstrual pads, you can make your own easily. Here's a pattern and instructions.

Maxi Pad
11.5 inches by
3.25 inches
approximately

First, cut a piece of 100% cotton flannel or fleece into this shape. Fold into the maxi pad and zigzag or serge around edges. Leave one edge finished but open to insert mini pad.

Mini Pad for heavy days. Cut 3 layers of cotton flannel or fleece into this shape. Zigzig or serge together. 8.75 inches by 2.75 inches approximately.

Sew Velcro to pad's bottom and to cotton underwear if you want to ensure no slippage - but cotton pad against cotton underwear is pretty secure.

Soak used cotton pads in water before washing. Wash in biodegradable soap, and if necessary, oxygen bleach. Tumble dry.

A mother can help a young woman enjoy her entry into puberty by directing her into appropriate womanly expression. Instead of rushing her into nylon stockings, unseemly makeup, and--of all things--training bras, a mother can teach a young girl to sew soft, colorful clothing out of cotton and silk, pleasurable fabrics that are healthy to wear. Many women are astonished to see their nervousness diminish and even disappear when they stop wearing synthetic fabrics. A girl can take pleasure from clean, flowing hair and healthy, rosy skin. Instead of pining away over images of skinny models and sexy movie stars, a girl can be led to emulate strong, healthy, vibrant women--perhaps their mother, perhaps their aunt--who are in harmony with themselves and with their environments, who love God, and who live joyfully and forcefully. Some girls thrive on school activities and plenty of interaction with peers, while others, more delicate in nature and spirit, need more quiet time, home time. Several teenage girls we know opened like flowers when they stopped attending public schools and pursued their studies in home school, only attending social activities as often as they felt like it. None of them developed into recluses as you might expect; in fact, after a period of time, each ventured into the world in her own way, one traveling to Europe, one becoming a nanny a continent away from her family, one apprenticing on a learning farm, and so on. How important it is for parents, especially mothers, to be quietly in tune with the needs of their daughters!

Puberty is a time to strengthen and tone one's body in preparation for parenthood. It is a time to run, to dance, to play ball, to jump and stretch and work hard at whatever activity pleases us. One modern dance teacher, pregnant at the time, told me that dancing well, training well, would help prepare my body for giving birth easily, and I found it to be so.

It is also a time to avoid anything that would weaken us. The controversy about marijuana and childbearing still rages; the active ingredient in the drug, tetrahydrocannibinol, crosses the placenta and also concentrates in breast milk, so a newborn can receive the cumulative effects of marijuana ingested by the mother. Proponents of taking the plant say that it is an herb like any other and cannot hurt anyone. However, no studies have been pursued to confirm either stance for sure. We feel that unhealthy substances, such as synthetic drugs, chemicals and so on, certainly have no place in anyone's system, but also that certain herbs can be inappropriate--including marijuana. We need to avoid anything that changes our clear, responsible perception of the world during the teenage years and throughout our lives.

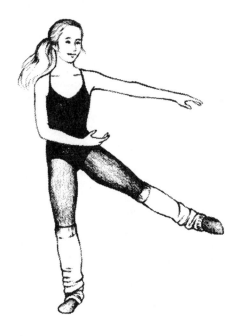

Many mothers have confided to me that during their teenage years they craved to hold, to be held. This was not a sexual longing so much as just a need for contact, for comfort. But in our society, few relationships permit this kind of holding, so a young girl's longing often leads her to sexual intimacy when she really didn't desire it, and wasn't ready for it. Fortunate is the girl whose family likes to hug, to touch, to hold. Even luckier is the girl who can help tend an infant or young child--an opportunity for plenty of hugging!

In a day where sexual intercourse is regarded as a physiological necessity, to be entered into as casually as going to the bathroom or having a meal, it almost seems anachronistic to restate Dr. Christopher's traditional views about morality. But even some medical doctors--Dr. Robert Mendelsohn, for example--consider that other issues of sexuality supersede the physiological. The moral, social, and spiritual aspects of sexuality affect us more profoundly than a new morality press would have us believe. How fortunate is the teenager whose parents can discuss sexual matters openly, without embarrassment, but most of all within a spiritual context. I suspect that more young people could avoid premature sexual contact if they could discuss the matter in a holistic way.

For a girl who takes plenty of exercise and uses the mucusless diet--including a gallon of water, preferably steam-distilled, every day, adolescence should offer no particular health problems. In fact, it should be the most healthy and happy time of her life!

But sometimes, especially if we are just beginning a cleansing and healing program, we experience problems. Very common is acne, which is most often a manifestation of an unclean bloodstream. Red clover tea is an excellent blood-cleanser, with a very mild taste. Burdock root tea works fast and well to cleanse the bloodstream. Carrot juice, very pleasant to the taste, cleanses and builds good cell structure. Many families drink green drink, consisting of fresh greens, such as comfrey, parsley, mint, lambsquarters, marshmallow (that is, common mallow), your dandelion and other local greens, blended into a base of pineapple juice in a blender. At first you may wish to strain out the pulp, but it is good for you too, and soon you should become accustomed to it. Some people make a green drink by simply blending the wildings into water, straining out the pulp and sweetening a bit with pure maple syrup or honey. This green drink supplies vitamins, minerals, enzymes, and healing factors in a fresh, assimilable form.

Don't forget the monthly three-day cleanse, which is a semi-fast. For three days you use no foods. Instead, you follow this simple program. Upon arising, drink sixteen ounces of prune juice--that's two cups--not only to cleanse the bowels but to purify the intestines. Then throughout the day, you drink one kind of juice, such as apple, carrot, grape, citrus, tomato, etc. Fresh raw juices are superior to canned, although good bottled grape juice has proven to be a good cleanser. Apple juice is a superior blood cleanser, too. You should use whatever is native to your area; if you live in an area growing citrus fruit, make up this combination: squeeze fresh in the morning four to six grapefruit, two to three lemons, and enough oranges to complete two quarts. Drink by swishing in the mouth before you swallow. Alternate whatever juices you drink with glasses of steam-distilled water. You should take about a gallon of juice in a day.

Don't eat anything during the day, although if you become very hungry towards night, you may eat an apple with the apple juice, carrot or celery with the carrot juice, etc.

During this juice fast, take one or two tablespoons of olive oil three times a day. This helps your liver take the toxins out of your body.

Be sure that your bowels are eliminating well during this time. If they aren't, take more prune juice, or take two or more capsules of Christopher's Lower Bowel Tonic, three times a day.

After your three-day cleanse, don't take a large meal. Instead, start eating a bit of fruit and nuts with your fruit juice, and then have a salad for lunch, including some raw vegetable juice. Repeat this for dinner; ease into more solid foods in the next day or two.

If you want to treat your acne externally, be aware that it's not an external problem. I would recommend very sparing use of soaps, which is contrary to most advice on acne. Soap removes the protective oil from the skin and upsets the acid-alkaline balance. Only use soap if your skin is really dirty; otherwise, wash with water. Instead of using thick makeup, which must be soaped off, let your natural healthy glow illuminate your skin. There are mineral-based blush powders which have no chemicals in them; they can be used as blush and as eyeshadow; just make sure when you purchase them that they really have no chemicals, as some cosmetic companies are mimicking the idea but including additives.

Some people recommend astringents to control large pores on oily skin. First of all, your skin won't produce excess oil if you follow the mucusless diet (see page 172). Although you will be taking adequate oils in your diet, they are in a form assimilable by the body. Probably the worst "junk food" anyone can take is hydrogenated oil--margarine, hydrogenated peanut butter, shortening. These oils have undergone a chemical change which makes their structures unusable by the body. They clog up the digestive tract and bloodstream and cause many problems, including that oily skin that troubles you! Eliminate them from your diet, replacing them with natural oils (olive, safflower, almond, sesame--there are many choices). You'll see a real difference in just about a week.

As for the large pores, astringents only help for a little while, as they fill the pores with moisture, seeming to close them. But after a short time, the pores return to their former size. A good diet, plenty of steam-distilled water, exercise, and the consistent use of the blood cleansing herbs mentioned above, will help tighten those pores. In the meantime (and perhaps just for fun) you can make some astringent lotions to apply to your face. Rub some strawberries on your skin and splash them away with water! Squeeze the juice from a cucumber and do the same. Tomatoes, raspberries, and zucchini all gently tone the skin. You can make a "green drink" for the complexion, blending comfrey, fennel, geranium, lavender, marigold, nettles, peppermint, sage or yarrow (any one or combination of these) with pineapple juice to make a thick mush. Put them on the face, containing them with a piece of gauze if necessary, and lie down for a half-hour or so. Rinse off and notice a glowing skin.

Good old-fashioned witch hazel (the distilled herb preserved with some alcohol), which you can still purchase at most pharmacies, is known for its skin-toning abilities. You can combine it with fresh or bottled (unsweetened) apple juice, adding a little rubbing alcohol to preserve. This fresh-smelling astringent is cheap enough for everyday use, but nice enough to bottle in a small container and give as a gift.

Dr. Christopher had many successes healing young women. One day a relative called him: "Do you want to see your favorite niece again? I don't think she's going to live until morning."

"Is Ann sick with asthma again?" Dr. Christopher asked.

"Yes," her father replied, "and the doctor doesn't think that she will survive it. Will you come out right away?"

"Sure, I'll see you just as soon as I can drive there."

"Oh, by the way," he said, as sort of an afterthought, "would you bring some herbs?"

Dr. Christopher smiled as he agreed, because this particular family didn't place much credence in his herbs. He didn't believe in running before he was called, even though he had seen this girl suffering with asthma for fourteen years; it was a family trait. Her father, although he knew that Dr. Christopher was an herbalist, had never asked his help. Dr. Christopher brought his wife with him, and went to their house.

Between the girl's gasps, he gave her sips of peppermint tea until she had taken a full cup. When she finished that, in about ten minutes, he gave her a teaspoonful of tincture of lobelia. In another ten minutes, he gave her another teaspoonful, and then a few minutes later, a third teaspoonful. He had never used more than three teaspoonfuls of the tincture of lobelia, because he was always called during asthma attacks at crisis. That is the best time to clear the ailment. They sat and talked after the girl had swallowed the third teaspoonful, and then she started to throw up. She vomited continually for an hour or so until she had nothing left in her; it brought up pus and phlegm from yellows to greens to blacks. She rolled over and fell asleep, so the Christophers left. She never had another asthma attack after that, as long as she stayed on the program, and grew up to have beautiful children of her own.

Another girl of fourteen had been born with polio, with one leg shriveled and four inches shorter than the other. She wore a built-up cork sole on her shoe, but she was still crippled.

The family read about Dr. Christopher's Incurables Program, and they began to follow it, step by step, for this girl. They used the Bone Flesh and Cartilage fomentation over that leg, continuing faithfully. By the time the girl was out of her teens, the leg was four inches longer than when she was fourteen years old. It was no longer shriveled; it filled out so it looked like the other leg. She was now dancing, and by the time she was in her early twenties, she not only ran her own dance school, but was demonstrating dance over the United States, traveling as a professional. The polio was gone. By going to the cause of the disease and working from there, we can cure even incurable diseases.

After a lecture, a woman came to ask Dr. Christopher to help her daughter, about fourteen years old, who tried to commit suicide. This girl required constant adult supervision to prevent her from harming herself. She had a skin disease diagnosed as being worse than psoriasis or anything else the doctors had seen. Scales covered her arms from the elbows down, her legs from the knees down, and her neck and face, with secondary bleeding. Having suffered with this for so many years, the girl could not attend school any longer, and was isolated at home. She gained tremendous excess weight, because in order to pacify herself, she would eat all day. Her mother called her a fat blob! And because she was getting worse and worse, she tried to kill herself.

As usual when presented with a difficult problem, Dr. Christopher offered a quick prayer, asking for guidance. The formula for the bone, flesh and cartilage combination (B F & C) came to him, step by step, and he told the woman to write it down. She wrote down all the herbs he mentioned, as well as the directions on how to put them together. She was to make a tea of six parts oak bark, three parts marshmallow root, three parts mullein herb, two parts wormwood, one part lobelia, one part skullcap, six parts comfrey root, three parts walnut bark (or leaves), and three parts gravel root. After soaking one ounce of the combined herbs in a pint of distilled water for four to six hours, she would simmer the mixture for thirty minutes, strain, and then simmer the liquid down to half its original volume. This could be made in larger amounts, whatever was needed. The mother would dip cotton flannel in this tea, or white cotton or wool stockings to cover the legs, with other long stockings to cover the arms. After covering all affected parts with these soaked cloths, she should wrap the arms and legs with plastic bags. This should remain on the girl all night, every night, until the morning. After a period of fresh air each day, the process would be repeated.

The mother tried this, and her daughter was very cooperative. The program began on a Tuesday, and although this disease had been worsening for many years, by Friday of that week all the scales had dropped off, and the skin was pink, healing.

After six months, when Dr. Christopher lectured in that city again, he learned that this young lady was back in high school, participating as a cheerleader, being very active. She was on the three-day cleanse and mucusless diet, as well as the red clover combination tea, the blood cleansers. Staying with this, she went from a large fat blob into a slender, well-shaped girl, overcoming her weight problem as well as the skin infection.

Once, when at a convention in the Northwest, a beautiful young lady came up to Dr. Christopher and his son, David. "How do you like my fingers?" she asked. They were well taken care of and the nails were done nicely. Dr. Christopher said, "Fine," and she asked, "Can you tell which finger has been cut off?" They couldn't tell. She showed him the finger that had been cut off; she used the B F & C combination, and the knuckle grew back, and the bone and flesh grew back in. The nail, which had been completely gone, grew back on, as pretty as the others. This was a truly unusual case of healing with the B F & C formula.

Here is an unusual case where Dr. Christopher used the B F & C formula on a young girl. He was lecturing in the Safford region of Arizona, and a man, who sponsored the lectures there, wished something could be done for his teenager daughter. They hated to sit down at the table with her, because she always scratched and picked at her head, digging the scabs out. The man brought her to where the lecture series was located so Dr. Christopher could take a look at her.

The girl had red hair, but there wasn't much of it. You could see her scalp, covered with sores which could not be cleared up. Dermatologists and other specialists could do nothing to stop the irritation on her head.

Dr. Christopher had her use the B F & C combination as a fomentation on her head. She soaked a cotton stocking cap--white, he emphasized, as herb combinations should never react with dye--with the concentrated B F & C formula tea, wearing this at night with a bathing cap over it. This would be left on all night, six nights a week.

After three months, Dr. Christopher lectured in the area again, and the girl came to show him that the scabs were all gone. Within the first week the itching stopped, and the sores healed up. But the hair that had been so thin was thickening, and by the time Dr. Christopher came back, she had a good head of hair, beautiful red and full as it had been years before.

Whether your teenage problems are serious, as these were, or minor, you can overcome them naturally with herbs and with a good diet. Living your teenage years happily and healthfully can help prepare you for bearing children and for doing a lifetime of significant and satisfying work.

BEFORE CHILDBEARING

Although the physical condition of both prospective parents affects the condition of a new child, the mother's health is most critical. Before conception, she and her husband should work together to purify and build their bodies in anticipation of pregnancy and childbirth.

So many factors influence the formation of a new child! It may take some time to build up the health of parents-to-be if they have been living on mucus-forming foods long before they marry.

If a young woman has menstrual problems, she can suspect that her female organs might not be in good condition. Although it should be needless to say, we should avoid drugs in managing our menstrual cramps. In order to treat the symptoms, some people favor red raspberry tea, peppermint tea, chamomile tea, ginger tea, or catnip tea. You can take a capsule of cayenne with any of these to help warm the internal organs. If the cramps are really severe, you can use a cayenne ointment such as Professor Cayenne's all natural Deep Heating Balm externally on the abdomen to act as a counter-irritant, but be sure to cover the application with gauze, as it can stain your underthings. Some young women have experimented with relaxation breathing, such as is taught in Lamaze childbirth classes. This allows the body to relax and deal with the pain, rather than fighting against it. Often tension really increases menstrual discomfort. Some women attribute cold in the abdominal region to the onset of cramps. Applying moist heat, such as a hot, moist towel covered with a piece of plastic, can help. If you wish to make an herbal fomentation of some of the pain-relieving teas mentioned above, it will even work faster and better.

One young woman wrote, "My sister and I suffered from menstrual cramps from the age of 13 on. We both started college at age 18. The first months after we started school, we noticed that neither of us experienced cramps anymore. The only thing we could attribute it to was the fact that we walked approximately 12 blocks to and from college classes five days a week. We are confident that the exercise did the trick. Up to that time, we just suffered it out." (*The People's Doctor*, Vol. 6, No. 7, page 3.)

As for the drugs you should avoid, knowing their effects may likely deter you from considering them as menstrual cramps panaceas. Aspirin, which can cause digestive-tract problems and deposit coal-tar traces throughout the system, actually doesn't work very well in relieving cramps. Tylenol, which has been the target for poisonings through tampering with the caps of bottles, offers its own dangers. It is evidently easy to overdose, which causes liver damage, sometimes resulting in death. Other effects are related to the liver, including jaundice and bleeding. Because the liver is the body's most important detoxifier, even small amounts of Tylenol may adversely affect the body's ability to handle toxins; these building up in the system may actually increase the pain in menstrual cramping! Talwin, a prescribed drug for the condition, causes nausea, dizziness and weakness and incapacitation. Birth control pills, which are sometimes prescribed for irregular and difficult menstruation, can cause abnormal bleeding and headaches, as well as sometimes endangering future fertility. Anaprox, which is a specifically-prescribed drug for menstrual pain, can cause headache, drowsiness, dizziness, lightheadedness, inability to concentrate, and depression. It can also cause skin reactions such as rash, sweating, easy bruising, and bleeding (Dr. Robert Mendelsohn, *The People's Doctor*, Vol. 6, No. 8).

In addition to avoiding drugs completely, one should be careful to avoid surgery for any kind of menstrual problems. Even if one's periods are irregular or if they stop completely, sometimes time and circumstances can alleviate the problem. If we are to follow the teachings of natural healers, surgery should be avoided except in the case of extreme, life-threatening emergencies for, as Dr. Christopher's Incurables Program has shown time and time again, even serious disorders can be healed naturally. Dr. Mendelsohn, cited above, suggested that sometimes sexual activity in marriage can produce the necessary hormones to activate a regular menstrual cycle. He also suggests that the clinical definition of menstrual normality should not frighten us, as some cycles are longer and some shorter than 28 days. In particular, we should avoid steroid drugs such as Prednisone, which really can cause problems with menstruation.

If a woman suspects that she has less than ideal function in her reproductive system, she can take red raspberry tea daily. She can also take Dr. Christopher's female corrective formula which rebuilds the entire reproductive area, and the hormone balancing herbal combination which will supply these factors in the correct amounts. They are present in a natural form, which allows the body to assimilate them as well as merely accept them. The female corrective formula consists of three parts golden seal root and one part each of the following herbs: blessed thistle, cayenne, cramp bark, false unicorn root, ginger, red raspberry leaves, squaw vine, and uva ursi.

Over the years, herbalists have helped women overcome painful menstruation, heavy flow, irregularity, etc. One woman in American Fork, Utah, was having difficult periods. These had started in puberty, and she had spent the whole of her adult life traveling from coast to coast, averaging a cost of over $1,000 a year for ten years, paying medical doctors to tell her what was wrong. She suffered vicious menstrual cramps and extremely long periods. No one was able to help; she was very discouraged; but one of her neighbors said, "Why don't you go to the next town, to Orem, where a man called Dr. Christopher lives? He could give you some help."

When she arrived, Dr. Christopher read her eyes, noting that she did have problems with the reproductive organs. He told her to start on the female corrective formula and the hormone balancing formula (which consists of black cohosh, sarsaparilla, ginseng, blessed thistle, licorice root, false unicorn root, and squaw vine). He promised her that if she would follow through, within 90 to 120 days she would get results. Within 120 days, she came back, saying that she was on a 28-day cycle, with no menstrual pains. She was delighted! Where she had spent over $10,000 traveling from doctor to doctor, it cost her approximately $10 for the herbs to cure her.

If you suffer from tumors or cysts in the reproductive organs, the herbal bolus (V.B.) formula has been reported to work wonders. Mix equal parts of squaw vine, slippery elm, yellow dock root, comfrey root, marshmallow root, chickweed herb, golden seal root, and mullein leaves. These should be powdered. Melt some coconut butter (solid at room temperature) and mix a small quantity of this powder in until it is of pie-dough consistency. Roll this between your hands until it is about the size of the middle finger and about an inch long. Insert several of these into the vagina, as you would use a suppository. You will need to wear a sanitary napkin. Leave in for two days; the coconut butter melts at body temperature, leaving only the herbs. On the night of the second day, douche with yellow dock combination herb tea cooled to tepid, and insert another bolus; after two more days douche again.

On the seventh day, you will rest. Repeat this pattern for six weeks to six months. This will bring out cysts, tumors, polyps, and acids through the vagina, through the rectum and the urethral tract.

A young Englishwoman named Claire suffered from multiple sclerosis so severely that she was confined to a wheelchair. She began to use the mucusless diet, and was miraculously healed and able to walk and work vigorously. Five women, each suffering from cervical cancer, diagnosed by doctors, came to Claire asking for help. Using nutrition and the herbal bolus therapy, four of the cases were completely cleared and one was in remission.

Sometimes it takes time and patience for these herbal aids to truly work. For example, a lady who had come to Dr. Christopher began the full routine as described above. A number of months later she began to think, "Look, I have been on that program for months now; I have taken the herbs orally; I've used the vaginal herbal bolus, including the yellow dock combination, and I am getting sick of this!" She felt somewhat better but didn't notice much change, so she was going to quit that day. That very morning she made the decision, as she was at home, sitting on the toilet. When she got up, she happened to turn around and glance into the bowl, and there was something about the size of a half dollar, with legs on it, swimming around in the water. This something had dropped out of her! She screamed, and her husband came in. They put it in a bottle and took it right over to the family doctor. He examined it under the microscope, and said he had never seen one of these whole like this, because they have to cut them out of a person. This was a spider cancer. They never give up and leave by themselves; usually they must be cut out. The doctor was amazed that it had come out of her. It had done so because her body was now so healthy that the spider cancer didn't have any waste materials to work on. When she saw that cancer, she vowed to continue the program, even if it took six months or years. Dr. Christopher reminded us that some people heal quickly, but sometimes it takes a long time. If we know we are on the right track, we should just continue.

If a couple wishes to delay conception for a time, perhaps in order to improve their health, they should be extremely cautious about what method of birth control they choose. Despite medical assurances that every method is safe, current research proves otherwise. Especially after taking birth control pills, some women suffer bad side effects, including infertility. According to Dr. Mendelsohn, this should not surprise anyone, because most of these pills suppress pituitary hormones because of the estrogenic and progestational hormonal activity of the ingredients in the Pill. The artificial hormones suppress the natural hormones in the body, leading to inhibition of ovulation as well as other effects. In addition to infertility, side effects may include abnormal bleeding and clotting, including cerebral hemorrhage and cerebral thrombosis. (*The People's Doctor*, Vol. 4, No. 1, page 5.)

According to information supplied by Planned Parenthood, each year 9,400 women are hospitalized because of complications from taking the Pill. Heart attack and stroke are the major culprits, causing about 500 deaths annually. About 11,000 women annually suffer from thrombosis (blood clots in the superficial veins). Liver tumors account for 300 annual hospitalizations, with a ten percent fatality rate. And 860 women are hospitalized annually for gall bladder problems caused by using the pill. Other complications which do not require hospitalization include nausea, breast enlargement, weight gain, dizziness, and liver spots on the skin. This same publication said that women who suffer from the following ailments must not take the Pill-- although the purpose of the booklet is to promote birth control use: phlebitis, stroke, coronary artery disease, benign liver tumor, and cancer of the breast or reproductive area. Women are also advised against taking the pill if they have high blood pressure, acute or chronic liver disease (and if the pill is so hard on the liver, it likely badly affects liver function to begin with), gall bladder disease, and those who are wearing long-leg casts or who have had a major injury to their feet or legs. Women who have diabetes or pre-diabetes (hypoglycemia?) and women expecting to have surgery should not take the Pill. ("Making Choices," Alan Guttmacher Institute, Planned Parenthood, 1983.) Considering all these problems and incipient health dangers, we would certainly advise no one to take the pill.

In addition, the insertion of an IUD may cause problems with conception. Dangers of using an IUD include abnormal bleeding, disturbances in menstrual cycles, fatal and non-fatal infected, spontaneous abortions if a woman becomes pregnant while wearing one, and perforation through the uterus and migration of the device into the abdominal cavity, which will require surgery. (*The People's Doctor*, Vol. 3, No. 12, page 3.) If a woman does become pregnant while wearing an IUD, she might bear children with birth defects. *The British Medical Journal* reported two women using copper-containing

IUDs who gave birth to children with malformation of the extremities, including missing fingers and toes, fused fingers, and reduced arm length. The article concluded that, while a relationship between birth defects and IUDs has not been conclusively proven, "the possibility of a relationship exists because of the proved association of IUDs with ectopic pregnancy, pelvic and fetal infection, miscarriage, premature labor, and fetal death" (quoted in *The People's Doctor*, op. cit.).

Although from Dr. Christopher's point of view, abortion certainly represents the most cruel kind of action, still many people are convinced by the medical world's claim that abortion is a good form of birth control. Doctors say that while in former times abortions were performed in unhygienic conditions, that today hospital abortions are perfectly safe. However, quite apart from the moral issue, which is really the paramount consideration anyway, consider this data from the *Journal of the American Medical Association:* "We compared prior pregnancy histories of two groups of multigravidas (women with more than one pregnancy)--240 women having a pregnancy loss up to 28 weeks' gestation and 1,072 women having a term delivery. Women who had two or more prior induced abortions had a two-fold to threefold increase in risk of first-trimester spontaneous abortion...The increased risk was present for women who had legal induced abortions since 1973. It was not explained by smoking status, history of prior spontaneous loss, prior abortion method, or degree of cervical dilation. No increase in risk of pregnancy loss was detected among women with a single prior induced abortion. We conclude that multiple induced abortions do increase the risk of subsequent pregnancy losses up to 28 weeks' gestation" (JAMA, June 27, 1980). In addition, research indicates that a previous abortion markedly increases the chance of temporary and sometimes permanent sterility (*The People's Doctor*, op.cit.). If you wish to bear children, do not submit to surgical murder via abortion. Indeed, it is better to avoid surgical intervention at all costs!

Suppose that a couple wishes to delay pregnancy, for health or other reasons. Delaying the birth of babies has become somewhat of a fad recently, and we do applaud any woman who conceives later in life and anticipates her baby with delight. Dr. Mendelsohn says that being fitted with a diaphragm is a safe method of contraception. Although it can be inconvenient, some couples use condoms. Midwives sometimes recommend the extended use of wild yam capsules. They say that it builds up contraceptive protection after being taken two or three months. These methods are preferred to the use of chemical applications such as foam, which is sometimes linked to cervical cancer.

But by far the most accurate and holistic approach to birth control was developed by John and Evelyn Billings during the late 1950's. This Australian couple--both doctors--were searching for a more effective alternative to the rhythm method, which doesn't always work. Reading anthropological literature of African and Indian tribes, they found a passing reference to the idea, "wet for baby, dry for no baby."

The Billings's asked the women in their charge to observe their vaginal discharges daily and to write down their observations. Virtually all the women noticed patterns in the changes of mucus production, and hormone tests confirmed that these changes were related to hormone changes.

Calling their discovery the Ovulation Method, the Billings's saw it taught to women in many Third World countries, in this way, "When the earth is dry and you plant a seed, it won't grow. When the rains come, the earth is wet and a planted seed will grow. For a few days after the rains, the ground is still wet, and a seed can still grow. When the ground is dry again, the seed will not grow when planted." Proven 98.5% effective, this method of birth control can also be an accurate way to achieve conception, so it is a very positive thing.

Basically, it works thus: The body's hormones develop several eggs, fully maturing only one. When this is released into the uterus, it lives for 12 to 24 hours, and if fertility were contingent only upon the presence of the egg, a woman could only conceive during that period of time. However, accompanying the production of the egg is the presence of fertile mucus. You might experience the cycle something like this. After your period, you might have days where your vagina seems quite dry. Then as your estrogen rises, you'll get wetter as you approach ovulation. When you ovulate, the wet or sticky secretion changes to a slippery one--that is fertile mucus. In the presence of this mucus sperm can survive; in infertile mucus, it dies, as the infertile mucus is extremely hostile to sperm. If a couple abstains from intercourse when the wetness first begins to appear, continuing to wait until three days after the slippery mucus appears, they are sure to avoid unwanted conception; or if they have intercourse during this fertile time, conception is more likely to occur. Why should the waiting period precede the actual ovulation? Because women have cervical crypts inside the vaginal passage, which can store sperm in a healthy condition until the body ovulates--as long as there is moisture. You may have heard of women who couldn't imagine that they conceived, because intercourse occurred several days before they reached the middle of their cycle--using the calculations of the Rhythm Method. However, the sperm was stored in the cervical crypts and traveled up the fertile mucus at the proper time.

This very brief description of the Ovulation Method will not suffice if you wish to use it yourself. *Mothering Magazine*, No. 37 (Fall 1985), supplies a good article on the subject; other good books include Terrie Guay's *Avoid or Achieve Pregnancy Naturally* (Emergence Publications, 1978), and *The Ovulation Charting Method* (Small World Publications, POB 305, Corvallis, OR 97339).

Dr. Christopher emphasized that many reproduction problems stem from the unkind and uncooperative behavior of husbands. He spoke openly to husbands who misused the privileges of marriage. For example, a certain woman came to Dr. Christopher in tears. Although the family had a number of children, she said life wasn't worth living any more because her husband forced her to have intercourse with him every night, whether she was sick, in pain, or pregnant. He said that if she wouldn't have intercourse with him, he would go out and get it someplace else, because it would damage his manhood if he didn't have it every night. She asked Dr. Christopher if this were true, that it would force a man into having other women. Of course, the woman was happy to learn that she did not have to suffer this kind of treatment; she said that she had gone through years of misery. After being forced for so long, she wanted some rest.

Dr. Christopher felt very strongly about this because he observed similar things in his own family. His own sister, now deceased, confided that her husband in Colorado demanded relationships every night; if she didn't give it to him, he would go up into town to a professional prostitute for relief. She said that she had suffered many nights of real sickness, yet allowed him to do this rather than have him leave home and go out with other women. The lady who adopted Dr. Christopher, who was the only mother he knew, also went through a similar trauma. As a teenager, he came downstairs to find his mother in tears. His adopted father had left, and the young Raymond asked what was wrong. In all the years they were married, she said, she had to satisfy her husband every night, "regardless of how sick I am." She suffered from arthritis and diabetes, sick through much of her life. Although some people might consider this an oddity, Dr. Christopher saw enough of it during his practice that he felt he must speak out on it. When such a situation occurs, he said, it is nothing but rape. Of course, sexual intercourse should be an exchange, a cooperation, an agreement, tender concern for the other person. Anything else Dr. Christopher considered rape, a disgrace.

In an age where millions of abortions are performed annually in the United States alone, it is an ironic tragedy that many childless couples long to conceive but cannot. Gynecologists sometimes go to great lengths to secure pregnancies for these couples, although the methods are not completely safe. As an example, Clomid, which is a fertility drug, causes flushes in ten percent of the women who use it, and ovarian enlargement in fourteen percent. Massive cystic enlargement of the ovaries may develop, a painful condition. The ovary continues to enlarge after the drug is discontinued, reaching its maximum size seven days after therapy stops! Other side effects include blurred vision, double vision, spots before the eyes, after-images, sensitivity to light, floaters, waves, cataracts, detachment of the posterior vitreous, spasm of the blood vessels, and thrombosis of the retinal arteries. A woman may also experience abdominal distention, bloating, abdominal or pelvic pain and soreness, nausea and vomiting, increased appetite, constipation, diarrhea, breast discomfort, abnormal menstrual bleeding, dryness of the vagina, headache, dizziness, lightheadedness, vertigo, nervous tension, insomnia, fatigue, depression, increased urinary frequency and/or volume, skin rashes, hair loss, hair dryness, weight gain or loss, jaundice, and fluid in the abdomen.

All of these possibilities would be bad enough, but the possible effects on an infant are worse. If a woman does not know that she is already pregnant and begins taking this drug, Clomid has been linked to congenital heart disease, Down's syndrome, clubfoot, congenital intestinal conditions, abnormal position of the urethral opening, small head, harelip, cleft palate, congenital hip displacement, birthmarks, undescended testes, extra fingers, conjoined twins, inguinal hernia, umbilical hernia, fused fingers, funnel chest, muscle disorders, dermoid cysts, spina bifida, and other defects. Most mothers who take the drug will have multiple births, usually -but not always- twins (*The People's Doctor*, Vol. 6, No. 11, p.6).

The other fertility drugs, such as Provera, Delalutin, or any other chemical substance designed to affect ovulation or fertility, present serious risks commensurate with these. A woman wishing to achieve a natural pregnancy cannot safely consider them.

One young mother, having difficulty with conceiving although she had previously borne two healthy children, went to a fertility specialist for help. The battery of tests--on both father and mother--revealed nothing really wrong, so the doctor gave her some medication without letting the woman know what she was taking. The fertility drugs produced a multiple pregnancy in the woman, and she bore triplets. Although the family was delighted to receive new little ones into the family, the multiple birth has been a tremendous strain on the family. Perhaps with more natural methods the family could have received their babies one at a time and with less stress and strain.

Dr. Mendelsohn suggests some basic approaches to conception, emphasizing the need to stay away from fertility drugs. He advises a nutritious diet, free of junk foods and additives, a sensible regular exercise program, an adequate amount of sleep and adherence to the marital requirements in the Old Testament. This law prohibits sexual intercourse during the menstrual period and for about a week afterwards. Not only does this time intercourse at appropriate fertility, but it also builds up the man's sperm so that there is better chance of fertilization. I feel that it also increases the health of the prospective mother, giving her female organs a chance to regulate themselves during her cycle.

Dr. Christopher had many successes helping couples conceive. One young married man came to see him about his wife, because he felt she was going to lose her mind. She wanted to have a baby so badly that she would hug her pillow at night. They had been married for some years without any success at conception. Dr. Christopher advised them to do the following: they should both begin to use the mucusless diet. In addition, they were to take two tablespoons of wheat-germ oil three times a day (this contains natural vitamin E;, among other constituents, which helps the reproductive system). They were to take two capsules three times daily of false unicorn and lobelia combination. If they were faithful with this program, the Doctor promised that they would conceive.

And they did! They brought the little baby in to see Dr. Christopher, and the new mother was absolutely glowing with health and joy at the baby in her arms. This couple had other children as well after following the simple herbal program.

Some couples have conceived when they have included more zinc in their diets, especially that of the father. When the problem is too-thick sperm (common in people on a mucus-causing diet), researchers have found that mega-doses of Vitamin C; (1000 mg. or more at each meal) has assisted in conception.

When couples marry and delay having children, they sometimes are tempted to continue on without having them. I can assure you that life without babies and children is much easier than with children! Nevertheless, I couldn't do without any of my children, and I don't begrudge them the time changing diapers, reading books, and tending them in the middle of the night.

Dr. Christopher taught much the same. He said that there are just so many babies that are supposed to be here on earth, and if we do our part, we will be able to take care of them. People who rear large families, and devote themselves to the families during their growing years, can do wonderful things. Dr. Christopher knew a family in Salt Lake City who had sixteen children, adopting the seventeenth. The man was only a clerk in an office, and you can imagine that they had a hard time making ends meet. Yet four of the sons became attorneys, a daughter became a professional dancer who demonstrates throughout the United States, and a son became a well-respected organist who performs throughout the country, and others of the children have accomplished great things. I know of a family with seventeen children, natural children in an intact family. Although the mother and father have to pour themselves out to nurture and teach that many, the older children participate in tending the younger ones, the home is well-cared-for and clean, and the children are well-disciplined. Of any baby-sitters I have ever had in my home, the oldest girls in that family have to be the best! They are intelligent and thorough and wonderful to be around.

In this day and age, most people are tuned into their own personal needs and consider childrearing a secondary sort of pursuit. What could be more far-reaching, however, than raising a whole, happy child? This extends to the third and fourth generation, to many other people than the child. And as for personal achievement, raising children has matured me, given me insights and capabilities that I never possessed before--and wouldn't have achieved without my little ones. I expect that when they are raised, I will be a much richer teacher and writer than I could have otherwise been, and having them has not stopped me from pursuing my career, albeit in a more limited way.

Dr. Christopher said that the children will be born, sometimes against our will! He remembered visiting with a family on business matters. The youngest child was one of the most positive and aggressive children he had ever seen. The mother would tell her to do something and the child said, no--she wanted to do it her way, even though she was still young. She had her own mind, and did what she wanted to do when she wanted to do it; nobody would push her around! Her father just laughed and said that the rest of the children were obedient and docile, except for this aggressive little child. He said that they had decided not to have any more children and his wife had an insert put in. The doctor assured them they wouldn't have any more. But months later, the wife found out she was pregnant. This child had decided that it would be their child regardless of the birth control method; the baby fought its way through and continued to be a fighter! The child was supposed to be there and made it safely. Dr. Christopher said that it sometimes pays just to let nature take its course.

Other herbs which have been used successfully to promote conception are red clover blossoms (these are considered by some to be as valuable as the false unicorn root), peppermint, stinging nettle, dong quai root, and of course red raspberry leaves.

If you are having difficulty ascertaining the timing of ovulation, or if your cycles are irregular, check to see if there is unnatural light interfering with your cycle. Sometimes when a street light shines in the window, or other lights are on all night, a woman's cycle can be really disrupted. Block out all unnatural light. Some practitioners have suggested that if women are quite irregular, they can keep a light on--say in the closet, or a mild night light--midway between periods, and that this will cause ovulation. A more natural, and more beautiful, alternative, is to sleep without the window shades, providing you live away from bright street lights. The light from the moon is thought to be healing and blessing; it can bring peace and regularity to your feminine cycle. Juliette de Bairacli Levy even suggests sleeping with no window screen--using an herbal insect repellent--to obtain maximum health. We have tried her repellent and it works. Here's how I made it: Combine equal parts of rue, wormwood, basil and rosemary. Grind in a mortar and pestle. Cover with about eight to ten times the herbs' volume of pure olive oil. You may add a couple of tablespoons of apple cider vinegar if you wish. Allow to stand in the sun--or over a radiator or other constant source of warmth--for a week. Strain out the herbs well, and repeat. Repeat a third time, this time letting the herbs stay in the oil as long as possible, perhaps up to three weeks. Although the time involved here is long, the actual work is minimal. Strain well and bottle. Although we have not tested this in terribly infested areas, such as jungle or summertime Alaska, it works for us during our summer camps. Levy said that she and her children slept outside in the Mexican tropical jungles, using this preparation, and were never bitten!

PREGNANCY

In spite of the morning sickness, aches and pains, and inconveniences pregnancy can cause, most women I know love to be pregnant. It is a time of heightened sensitivity, of blossoming. Pregnancy is a time of health, not of disease, and so we should treat ourselves not as patients but as women acting out an important part of our life's drama. This can be difficult if we consult a doctor who treats us as though for disease. I consider a woman's choice of prenatal care of utmost significance.

What you do during your pregnancy can make all the difference to your birth experience. Medical doctors admit that prenatal nutrition and exercise vitally affect the birth process and health of the newborn. One (very enlightened) M.D. said that he'd rather see a lady eat and exercise truly well--and then be knocked out with drugs for the birth--rather than see a woman during pregnancy fill herself with junk food and drugs and seek a natural birth. He might be exaggerating a little, but you owe it to your baby and yourself to do the very best you can during pregnancy.

If you follow the mucusless diet during your pregnancy, you will be able to supply your baby everything it needs for good development. The general idea is to avoid any processed food and to concentrate on fresh, live foods that will digest well and give both of you what you need. If you feel you need more protein during gestation, try sprouting some sunflower seeds. They taste delicious in salad and provide an excellent quality protein. Sprouted almonds are said to be a perfect protein. Dr. Christopher suggested soaking dried beans (such as pinto, etc.) for 24 hours, then low-heating them for a day or two. Seasoned with garlic, tomatoes, basil, oregano, and chili powder, these beans are delicious and really satisfying. Unseasoned, you can mash them in a hot pan with a little oil, adding water as necessary to make a creamy consistency, for really good refried beans. This provides a digestible and satisfying protein.

Be very careful with dairy products, as they create mucus in most people. Raw milk is better than pasteurized; yogurt (homemade) is better than raw milk; goat's milk is better than cow's milk. However, butter is much better than margarine, although you can use cold-pressed oils for your fat needs. Margarine is made from hydrogenated oils, which are indigestible and coat the intestinal tract and bloodstream.

One nutritionist called it the worst junk food he knew of. You may eat cheese sparingly, but concentrate on the vegetarian sources of protein.

People who eat meat might try to be sensitive as to the kinds and amounts taken during pregnancy. We honor the kosher law which forbids pork, shellfish, and various other kinds of unusual meats (see Deuteronomy 14:3-21). Many also warn against consuming too many red meats. They are much heavier, and most of them have received strong doses of chemicals, including stilbestrol to induce growth. Many such treated red meats have been suspected of a relationship with cancer. Probably the best meats are homegrown chickens and fish from clean waters. Remember to use them only "in times of cold or famine."

As for cravings, having been a pregnant woman, I feel it is right to feed your craving as long as it is a good wholesome food. Sometimes we break the rules when the craving is intense; during a couple of pregnancies, I badly wanted to eat potato chips! We got some at a health-food store and I felt better after eating them. Many women crave berries, and this is appropriate, because berries feed nutrients into the system that our bodies may be crying for. One prenatal adviser suggested using berries from the area in which we are born and raised; some of us in the West crave raspberries, where they abound; some from the East and Northwest crave blueberries. Strawberries may satisfy an Eastern or Californian expectant mother. If you are going to be pregnant during the winter, obtain some good, organically-grown berries, wash them and pat them dry, and freeze them whole in rigid-sided containers in your freezer. You may use them almost-thawed during the winter, or blend them into smoothies with juices or soy or nut milk. They keep their quality very well.

During my fifth pregnancy, we camped for three months in the Alaskan wilds. Living primitively, we carried with us seeds, nuts and grains, used some grocery produce (terrifically expensive!) and local produce. Out in the muskeg where we camped abounded incredible amounts of wild blueberries; we ate blueberries all sorts of ways--in cobblers, cooked with a little honey, in pies, over cereal--you name it! We also ate some Alaskan salmon cooked over the fire. Combined with the 24-hour day (no night during the summer in Alaska) and exposure to the sun, air and earth--and perhaps some genetic contribution--this fifth baby weighed nine and a half pounds when he was born, compared to our usual seven-pound newborns! I have to give some credit to blueberries.

From conception, I recommend taking the following herbs either in green drink or in tea. They seem to me to be the best pregnancy combination possible: equal parts comfrey leaf, raspberry leaf, and alfalfa leaf. During the summer, blend these with enough pineapple juice (in a blender) to make a drinkable mixture. Use a few ice cubes or a little water to thin the mixture if you wish. During the winter, mix the herbs and make a standard infusion. Sweeten with honey and drink at least a quart a day, more if you like it. You can make it into cool tea in the refrigerator if preferred. This provides nutrients and medicinal factors that are necessary for a good, strong pregnancy. Raspberry leaf tea has been proven to contain fragarine, a medicinal constituent proven to assist in pregnancy and birth (Grantly Dick-Read, *Childbirth Without Fear,* New York: Harper & Brothers, 1959, p. 211, note). Red raspberry contains citrate of iron in an assimilable form, a wonderful source of iron for expectant mothers. The comfrey is a cell proliferant and provider of a variety of minerals and enzymes. The alfalfa is a wonderful mineral source as well as providing lots of Vitamin K;, which helps in blood clotting.

MORNING SICKNESS

If you should suffer from morning sickness you, like the rest of us, may feel overwhelmed by the severity of the symptoms. I had planned our sixth pregnancy, and for months before had worked to build up my adrenal glands, as I had read that adrenal exhaustion can worsen morning sickness. I was concentrating on a good diet, and walking and running up and down the foothills near our home. I was also taking at least a quart of red raspberry leaf tea daily. With this program, I thought I would be sure to mitigate the nausea and vomiting.

Two or three weeks after conception passed--no nausea. I had conquered! And then one day I woke up nauseated and vomiting. Whatever hormonal mechanism that triggers the problem had occurred, and I suffered my usual three-month ordeal of morning sickness. Some women benefit from Vitamin B-6 treatment during this time: they take 200 mg. for seven days and five mg. per day thereafter as long as the problem persists--which is usually to the beginning of the fourth month. I cannot say that B-6 ever helped me much! Some women have said that ginger capsules have alleviated the nausea (ginger has been proven to be more effective for travel sickness than Dramamine, the over-the-counter drug). I have made ginger ale at home, supplying some relief. Here is how it's done:

Heat a gallon of water quite warm, enough to dissolve 1 cup of honey and to release the flavor of 2 tablespoons of ginger. Add these and let cool somewhat, until lukewarm. Add the juice of four lemons, mix well, and then stir in 1/4 teaspoon of baking yeast. Put into a gallon jar, cover lightly, and let sit for about 24 hours. If you wish, you can strain, but we just pour it off the top and discard the dregs when we're done. Refrigerate to enhance the sparkle and stop fermentation. Drink as required to help with nausea. I wonder which helps most, the ginger or the honey, as some practitioners assert that morning sickness is a blood-sugar problem. The baby takes the mother's nourishment, leaving her hypoglycemic and unable to easily recover.

This may be true, but during this pregnancy my morning sickness was helped most by a mineral preparation called Body Toddy that someone gave me. By following directions I was able to stop vomiting, although the nausea continued, somewhat abated, until the usual time. Another excellent remedy for minerals is powered barley leaves, which helped me a lot during one pregnancy. Perhaps the body calls for minerals as well as more consistent nourishment during this time.

Some expectant mothers get results with teas of basil, red raspberry, peach leaves, or one of the mints. Be careful not to overtake your favorite tea during this time, or you may not be able to stomach it for the rest of your life! This sounds ridiculous, but often the smell or taste of a food taken during times of morning sickness can bring back the nausea long after the baby is born. During one pregnancy, my small children played a particular record, "Winnie the Pooh." To this day, whenever I hear this record, I feel sick to my stomach! We ate corn on the cob and fresh trout during my first pregnancy, and I still can't eat the combination without a touch of queasiness. This is not to say that I consider morning sickness a mental affliction; after going through it six times I assure you it is quite real. Probably the best remedies I could recommend are exercise in the fresh air, and something interesting and active to do during this period. After nine pregnancies, I have concluded that emotional stress (centered in your stomach) may strongly exacerbate morning sickness. If you can manage a short, stress-free vacation --perhaps alone-- during the morning sickness months, you may be able to overcome some of the nausea.

Some herbalists consider that chemical by-products of the hormonal changes in the body may cause morning sickness. You should walk at least a mile a day to eliminate these toxins, and try to avoid adding toxins to your system by wrong eating. The daily green drink is a good way to supply fresh chlorophyll into your body to prevent toxic build-up.

By all means, do not take any drugs, prescription or otherwise, to alleviate the symptoms of morning sickness. During the last twenty-five years the drug Bendectin has been routinely prescribed for morning sickness. It has finally been taken off the market by its manufacturers because of its devastating effects: foreshortening of the extremities and absence of fingers and toes. Pyloric stenosis, a closing off of the outlet of the stomach which sometimes requires surgery in babies, is also linked to the drug; babies with pyloric stenosis are four times as likely to have been exposed to Bendectin. There is also an increased risk of gastrointestinal malformations, especially failure of the esophagus to develop and failure of part of the intestinal tract to develop in infants of mothers who were prescribed Bendectin.

The manufacturer, Merrel-Dow, has withdrawn the drug from the market, not because of these dangers, but because it cannot keep up with the $1 million monthly liability insurance necessary to defend itself against lawsuits. The company has sent letters to doctors assuring them that they will try to maintain current supplies of Bendectin anyway so that current patients can continue this "therapy." In other words, even though research has indicated that birth defects are connected with the drug, the manufacturer would continue to supply it if they could get away with it! At the very least, we can refuse to take it!

Sherry Lynn Mims Jiminez suggests that "this temporary condition of morning sickness can occur in pregnancy due to the excessive protein requirements of the developing fetus." She suggests neutralizing stomach acids by eating an apple or potato without the peel. She also recommends the old-time remedy of soda crackers. Frequent snacks of protein-rich food are said to help (from *The Pregnant Woman's Comfort Guide*, Prentice-Hall, 1983).

If you move around slowly, you can sometimes avert an onset of morning sickness. Some women get relief from eating crackers or matzo first thing in the morning. Greasy or fried foods may nauseate you, although sometimes I simply crave fried things; during my last bout of morning sickness we ate fried whole-wheat scones once or twice a week; the fried bread was what my body craved! Apple-cider vinegar and honey may take the edge off your nausea.

Most women get over the morning sickness when they hit the four-month mark in pregnancy. The only sure cure, in most cases, is time, but for those unfortunate mothers-to-be who feel nauseated during most of their pregnancy, I would suggest trying some of these methods and perhaps visiting a natural-healing practitioner to ascertain the cause for the ongoing nausea.

The second trimester of pregnancy--four to six months--can provide great joy to the mother-to-be. You have seen happily pregnant women; their faces fill out, their cheeks glow, and their eyes shine with an unusual light. Many women get a real thrill at the changes in their bodies, the growing breasts, the rounding belly. If the husband is gentle, pregnancy can be a fine time for lovemaking, as there's no concern about getting pregnant! An expectant mother should continue her comfrey-raspberry-alfalfa tea, a good diet, and a daily walk. I feel that the walk has prepared me for birthing as much as any other practice. It tones the muscles and gives oxygen to mother and baby. It also cheers you up! If there are other children in the family, perhaps the father can tend them during this time so the mother can enjoy a good brisk walk alone, a time for meditation and prayer. My husband has done this for me during all of my pregnancies, and I have treasured it as a quiet, personal gift.

WEIGHT GAIN

As long as the mother-to-be is following the mucusless diet, she should not concern herself about weight gain. Where doctors formerly warned women not to gain more than ten or fifteen pounds, it is now acceptable to gain thirty or forty during a pregnancy. This can be difficult for women who are enculturated to appreciate skinniness and abhor round, full bodies. Rather than emphasizing calorie intake, I would just recommend eating plenty to satisfy your appetite, tuning in carefully to what your body is asking for. Completely avoid any processed foods, preparing what you eat at home according to the guidelines of the mucusless diet (see page 172). Sometimes pregnant women develop ravenous hunger--lactating women do, too. Enjoy a variety of foods in your diet, always emphasizing those foods that grow in your area as opposed to foods imported from long distances away. Some women who have trouble relaxing and gaining adequate weight for pregnancy have suggested visualizing themselves beautiful, round and full during pregnancy, or sewing themselves a maternity dress that they can wear after they have gained ten pounds. If you are following the mucusless diet, you will be supplying good building materials for your baby. Remember that you are also building a necessary fat supply to help nurse your little one.

TECHNOLOGY

Many women under the care of an obstetrician are faced with worse problems than bad advice on weight gain. Nowadays doctors routinely apply certain techniques to pregnancy that are extremely questionable. For example, many women undergo amniocentesis, which draws fluid from the uterus; the fluid is then analyzed. This technique can reveal the baby's sex (for those family planners who want only one child of each sex), and if the sex is undesired the mother is given the option of abortion! This is a red-hot moral issue, and any naturally-oriented mother will avoid the technique absolutely. If a defective child is diagnosed, such as one who is Mongoloid, the mother can also choose to abort. Yet the laboratory tests are not always certain, standing a fifteen percent chance of being inaccurate (*The People's Doctor*, Vol . 3, No. 11). The dangers of amniocentesis include air in the baby's chest from being punctured with the needle introduced to extract fluid, gangrene of a fetal limb from the same, hemorrhage, and sudden fetal death Even if a problem is diagnosed, the options are not simple: either abortion or the possibility of spending the rest of one's life caring for a sick or disabled child. "When we talk to women now in their 50s and 60s about the children they bore while in their 30s and 40s, they do not talk about the fear of Down's syndrome haunting their pregnancies. That is not to say that they were not indeed at some risk, only that it was not constantly being brought to their attention....For the 99 or so out of 100 40-year-old women of earlier generations who bore children without Down's syndrome, ignorance may have been, if not blissful, at least relatively peaceful." (Barbara Katz Rothman, "The Selling of Amniocentesis," *Mothering*, No. 37, Fall 1985, p. 77.)

More subtle, but potentially more dangerous, is the routine application of ultrasound in normal pregnancies. Although most medical practitioners assure us that ultrasound presents no dangers, this procedure, which is used to study the body's internal organs with non-ionizing waves, has been the subject of research indicating some considerable risks. Although supposedly said to work with sound waves, they are not in the audible range, so their high frequency is not natural to the body. Dr. Mendelsohn wrote, "Ultrasound produces at least two biological effects--heat and a process called 'cavitation' in which bubbles are created that expand and contract in response to sound waves. The first time I saw this cavitation process in action, a chiropractor turned on the therapeutic ultrasound machine in his office and placed a few drops of water on the part of the machine that was applied to the patient. I wish every reader...could have been with me to watch that water suddenly boil and bubble" (*The People's Doctor*, Vol., No. 11, p. 3).

After ferreting out the truth about ultrasound over the years, Dr. Mendelsohn received copies of documents researching the procedure, which anyone may receive by writing *WHO* Publications Center, 49 Sheridan Ave., Albany, NY 12210, asking for "Environmental Health Criteria 22: Ultrasound." Experiments cited in these documents indicated reduced fetal weight and reduced fetal organ weight in animals who received ultrasound. Researchers are noticing a small but definite reduction in newborn birth weight among human infants exposed to ultrasound. The immune systems of laboratory animals exposed to the procedure are said to be affected. It also affects the blood platelets which allow the blood to clot. This could lead to problems with circulation because of traveling blood clots. Changes in the structure and composition of cells, including genetic material, has been suspected. In experiments with animals, these changes have resulted in defective embryos with a variety of problems. Researchers postulate that problems incurred by ultrasound could take as long as 20 years to surface, including the possibility of cancer and, most commonly suspected, leukemia. The mother might also experience congenital malformations.

The experiments on animals don't necessarily prove that humans will suffer in exactly the same way. But, as Mendelsohn points, when animals were tested with Thalidomide, the anti-nausea drug freely administered during the first decades of this century, animals did not show the terrible skeletal deformities that humans suffered.

Ultrasound has never been proven to beneficially affect the outcome of pregnancy either for the mother or the newborn. Researchers indicate that only in cases of definite risk should ultrasound be administered. Why do most doctors give ultrasound? To check the development of the baby--to ascertain position of the baby--to check for twins--to see where the placenta is placed--to check the size of baby's head--and so on. Most times the baby's sex is announced, which deflates some of the delightful mystery of giving birth.

Along with other medical doctors, Mendelsohn suggests that ultrasound falls into the same category as the frequent use of X-rays during earlier years. At that time no one knew how dangerous X-rays could be; even shoe salesmen used fluoroscopes to see if shoes fit the feet properly! He says that mothers-to-be should absolutely avoid ultrasound during normal pregnancy. And we should be careful about the too-frequent assignment of the rating "high-risk" pregnancy. I was astonished that I was among that category, in my mid-thirties and having borne six children. My health is excellent and my births are fast and straightforward. Only on the strength of several opinions--perhaps including a good lay midwife--should anyone submit herself to a now routine practice that may eventually prove dangerous. And, as Mendelsohn also advises, if you and your baby have already exposed to ultrasound, you should obtain all medical records of the procedure, so that if some tragedy should develop in the future, you will have proof.

Realize too that the Doppler stethoscope uses ultrasound to detect fetal heart rate. One should insist on the traditional fetal stethoscope.

It should go without saying that a mother-to-be should avoid examination by X-ray unless there is some mortal danger involved. Even tooth X-rays should be avoided. Interestingly, some dental technicians are very sensitive to risks presented pregnant women; one technician rescheduled a tooth cleaning session for me until after the birth, wishing to avoid introduction of bacteria caused by the cleaning. X-rays have been associated with cancer and genetic abnormalities.

In fetoscopy, the doctor looks at the fetus as a needle and small telescope-like instrument are inserted through an incision near the pubic bone into the uterus, allowing a view of the fetus. Possible hazards include damage to the fetus' eyes from too intense a light, as well as possible miscarriage, premature labor, and hemorrhage.

Other interventions, such as non-stress tests, chorion biopsy, where samples of the outer fetal membrane are extracted and analyzed, or the contraction stress test, which temporarily induces labor and checks the fetus' ability to handle the contractions, are variously dangerous and have not been proven to be helpful. And as we show in the following chapter, monitoring during labor presents real risks as well.

If all these medical interventions are dangerous, what can parents do to ensure a safe pregnancy and birth?

Maybe the answer seems too simple: the daily use of the three-herb tea or green drink, red raspberry, comfrey and alfalfa; the careful adherence to the mucusless diet; adequate exercise in the fresh air; at least a gallon of distilled water daily. Many midwives swear by the daily sitz bath, which is taken by immersing the bottom and abdomen in a wash tub of very warm water for about a half hour every day. This softens and tones up the pregnant bottom and relaxes the mother. If you don't have a wash tub, you can take a sitz bath by propping your feet up on the end of the tub and soaking your lower parts; then take a bath as usual. At least switch from showers to baths during pregnancy so you can enjoy the relaxing and detoxifying effects.

EXERCISE

Perhaps one of the most neglected aspects of pregnancy is exercise. Especially during the period of morning sickness, the prospective mother feels like doing nothing, and her exercise program often goes by the board for the rest of the pregnancy. If you actively participate in some exercise before conception, you can continue with it virtually throughout your term, although I found I needed to switch from jogging to fast walking at about six months. However, tennis, horseback riding, dance--whatever you do can be continued as long as you feel comfortable doing it. If you begin to feel too heavy to do some aspect of the activity, still you can continue to do what you can. Don't stop! Swimming is one of the best activities for pregnant women; the water buoys the belly up, the whole body is exercised, and it can be continued right up until birth. One friend in her early forties, carrying her second child, swam on the day she went into labor!

Some special exercises have been developed by various people to continue through pregnancy. Jane Fonda has produced such a series. You may be able to locate something appealing in your public library.

Here are some tried-and-true standard exercises that might help you during pregnancy.

When you bend down, always squat rather than bending over. When you sit on the floor, sit in Indian fashion, or tailor position. Spend a good deal of time sitting this way on the floor--in either position. This tones up the birthing muscles.

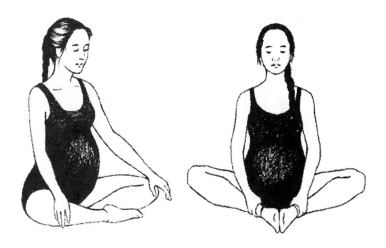

Sit on the floor with the soles of your feet touching, your knees out. Press your knees toward the floor, not stretching too much, but pulling and stretching the inner thigh muscles. This is a dance exercise I learned before I was married, and it is excellent for toning up the inner thighs, which sometimes lock up during birth.

Kegel exercises may be performed anytime in a woman's life, but are especially helpful during pregnancy. From a relaxed feeling in the vaginal floor, draw up the muscles as if you were stopping urination. Pull them up tight, and then relax them again. Repeat many times throughout the day. No one can tell you are exercising as you do the Kegel's while standing in line, sitting at your desk, cooking or wherever. Not only does this tone the birth canal, it strengthens your lovemaking muscles, and some couples report more pleasure after a woman has conscientiously done Kegel exercise.

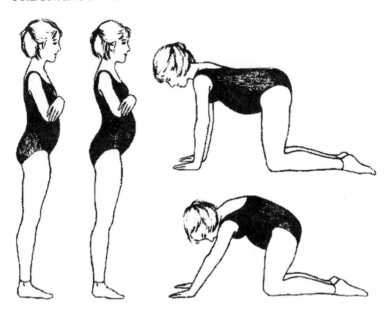

The pelvic rock is a standard prenatal exercise. On your hand and knees, arch your back clear up, then let it sag clear down. Repeat as needed. This can help a baby's position, but it also feels wonderful to an aching mama.

From a good, straight standing position, rock your pelvis back so that your belly falls forward and your bottom sticks out. Return to the original position and repeat several times. This strengthens the muscles of the lower back, which really take a beating during pregnancy and afterward, when you carry the baby around.

These standard pregnancy exercises are a good beginning; you can supplement them with modifications of regular calisthenics. Do a partial sit-up several times, repeating as desired. Remember the cross-touching-toes exercise from school days, when you bend over spread feet and touch your right toe with your left hand, etc. You won't be able to reach your toes, perhaps, but this is a good limbering and toning exercise. Knee bends, done slowly, are a variation of the squat, which are marvelous for keeping your legs and hips toned and trimmed. Slow, thorough arm circles are excellent. If you are into Yoga, you might look up a book on Yoga in pregnancy.

Although carrying a child is a spiritual and emotional experience, it is first of all a physical one, and what you do physically strongly influences the way you feel in other ways.

You may experience some of the usual problems during pregnancy, and herbs-- combined with other natural practices--can help you get over these.

CONSTIPATION

Some women get constipated during the first trimester; this is because the intestinal action is slowing down. That is why you may gain weight faster than you think you should; your intestines are absorbing more from the food you eat. Here are some suggestions to improve elimination. Eat more raw food, especially apples and carrots. Take more liquid in your diet, not only water, but soup, smoothies made with fruit, brewer's yeast, and yogurt, juices, teas. Exercise more, especially uphill running or walking. You can take bran or psyllium seed in water. Chia seed blended into a smoothie helps elimination and provide wonderful nutrition. You can take prune juice or eat prunes. Violet leaves are gently laxative. You may take one or two capsules of Dr. Christopher's lower bowel formula, but generally be careful of laxatives, even herbal ones. The lower bowel formula is a bowel toner and healer, and does not offer the same problems as many herbal laxatives, but please use it with prudence. First use fruits and vegetables that provide wholesome fiber as a laxative.

ANEMIA

Anemia may be caused by iron deficiency or other problems. Iron supplements are commonly given to expectant mothers, yet these are usually made of ferrous sulphate and cannot be utilized by the body. Being inorganic, they are absorbed but not assimilated and can cause problems in the system. In addition, they destroy vitamin E that may be taken at the same time. You can build up the iron in your system by taking yellow dock or the yellow dock combination. Some midwives say that yellow dock alone doesn't help for very long; its effect sometimes wears off. I have had excellent results combining yellow dock root and dandelion root; dandelion contains an excellent spectrum of minerals that enhance the 40% iron content of the yellow dock. Some good iron-containing foods include apricots, sunflower seeds, black molasses, raisins, prunes, brewer's yeast, kelp, egg yolk, grains, beets and their greens, turnip greens, dulse, and walnuts. If you do not respond to the dietary additions here, suspect folic acid anemia. Many pregnant women are woefully under-supplied with folic acid, and although you can get a prescription for folic acid supplements, this fragmented source may not be well absorbed by your body. Better to obtain this important nutrient in foods; some important sources are whole grains, leafy greens, watercress, parsley, chicory, dandelion, amaranth, and lambsquarters. Some of these can be taken in the green drink; lambsquarters is especially valuable as it also contains a large amount of vitamin A which helps prevent infections.

INDIGESTION

Many women experience indigestion and heartburn, and sometimes gas, during pregnancy. This may be caused by the stomach having less room to do its work, nervous tension which inhibits good digestion, too many stomach acids, or a relaxed stomach, which allows foods to back up. Be sure that you do not take antacids during pregnancy. They further inhibit digestion, and they may cross over the placenta into the baby. To deal with these symptoms, Dr. Christopher first emphasized that we must chew our food. Many of us just gulp it down, and the large particles cause gas, fermentation, and pain. Chew well; even juices should be swished in the mouth to mix them with saliva and begin digestion. Don't drink with your meals; water or other liquids dilute the digestive fluids. You may, however, want to take broth or juices with the meal, but you should "chew" these too. Increase your B-vitamin foods, including whole grains, brewer's yeast, wheat germ, yogurt, perhaps acidophilus. Don't smoke or drink tea or coffee; these irritate the stomach and increase heartburn. Eat small meals frequently. If you must be away from home, take juice, fruit and nuts with you to prevent your blood sugar going down and stomach acids overproducing. Papaya can aid digestion--fresh, dried or in tablets. Some women take tablets of activated charcoal to absorb gases in the system. Slippery elm gruel will alleviate heartburn and absorb gases and toxins.

BACKACHE

If you get a backache, try the pelvic rock exercise (unless your toddler climbs up on your back!). Don't lift heavy objects, and never bend over, letting the weight of the abdomen pull on your back; always squat. Don't wear high-heeled shoes; low heels are best, and shoes like Birkenstock sandals or Earth Shoes are wonderful for relieving pressure in the back. I had real foot and back pain until I bought myself a pair of Birkenstocks; the pain went away right away. Sitz baths can alleviate backache. You may need a chiropractic adjustment. Find a practitioner who understands the strains of pregnancy and who is not just a bone-cracker, but who can help balance the muscles that hold the vertebrae in place. You can place pillows behind your back or at your belly to avoid muscle strain when you sleep. Some companies sell a body-sized pillow to wrap yourself around and alleviate pressure during sleep -a real luxury, but wonderful if you can afford it. Take Dr. Christopher's calcium formula to make sure you have enough calcium and related minerals to relieve the pain and nourish the muscles. Some women have taken wheat-grass juice; the concentrated chlorophyll has been used to remedy backaches. Plant soaked wheat seeds in a seed flat filled with dirt. Water each day and when the shoots begin to look like grass, several inches high, you can cut them. The best way to obtain the juice is to put them through a special wheat-grass juicer, but if you haven't got one, blend the grass with water in your blender, strain, and drink. Sometimes backaches are caused by kidney problems, which you can treat by taking lemon water, nettle tea, or using Dr. Christopher's kidney and bladder formula. You can rub Professor Cayenne's Deep Heating Balm, Olbas or other heat-inducing ointments on the back to relieve pain. Your husband may be able to press the sore spots firmly but gently and relieve much of the stress.

MUSCLE PAINS

Some women get persistent or shooting pains down their thighs, especially during the last part of pregnancy but often earlier. These pains are caused by the baby pressing on the related nerves, but during the last part of pregnancy, they are the result of the baby pressing its head against the os, trying to soften it up, getting ready for birth--a nice sign however painful! Use some of the above treatments to help relieve this muscle pain. The best approach, however, is to lie down and have your husband or someone else press the muscles inside the thighs and between the hip bones and the pelvic bones. You should be able to locate many very tight muscles all along these areas. Press them quite firmly until the tightness disappears, and you will notice a marvelous relaxing throughout the body, relieving not just the muscle spasms, but all sorts of tensions you might not have been aware of before. This treatment cannot damage mother or baby, so repeat it as often and as hard--within reason--as desired. This is also good for the dreadful aching some women get throughout the crotch area, especially in multiparas.

VARICOSITIES

Varicose veins and hemorrhoids are both evidence of the same problem: lack of nutrients causing weakness in the circulatory system. Improving the diet and supplementing with the calcium formula makes a big difference in the problem right away. One woman who suffered from large, painful varicosities in the legs took Body Toddy, a liquid mineral preparation, and the swelling and varicosities themselves eventually disappeared. Dr. Christopher recommended making a strong tea of oak bark, soaking cotton stockings in it, and applying these over the affected parts. This should clear the varicosities easily. If you are suffering from hemorrhoids, a sitz bath of strong oak bark tea will help, as well a Sitz of witch hazel tea. You can apply drugstore witch hazel on the hemorrhoids. Make an ointment of comfrey or yellow dock for the area. We have had good results with plantain and mullein ointments. Dr. Christopher suggested inserting a piece of red potato, about the size of the little finger, into the rectum, for nearly instant relief. Certain factors in the diet certainly cause hemorrhoids--junk foods of all kinds can clog up the circulatory system. For a couple of weeks, we tried using the cheaper margarine instead of our usual butter. After that time, we experienced large, protruding and very painful hemorrhoids, as well as congestion generally. When we began using butter and oil again, the symptoms just disappeared. This confirmed the belief that margarine is a dangerous junk food! The body cannot handle the hydrogenated oils. Although our experience flies in the face of standard dietary recommendations, which say that butter is dangerous, not margarine, we think that a moderate amount of butter is fine.

If you get irritated, itchy skin on your belly, rub it regularly with coconut oil or olive oil, which may be scented with natural flavor oils. Be aware, however, that these oils stain cotton underthings a nasty gray--permanently.

URINARY INFECTIONS

Sometimes women get urinary infections if they are subjected to stress or unusual toxicity or other infections. From personal experience, I can tell you that you must attend to these right away, or they can become extremely painful and make you very sick. You should drink as much fluid as you can, in the form of teas, water, and juices; beware of too much sweetness, however. Cranberry juice is the standard remedy, but this must be unsweetened, usually obtainable from the health food store, or made on your juicer at home. It is sour, not nearly as pleasant as the bottled grocery store variety. Use the herbal kidney and bladder formula found in the formulas section at the back of this book. Yarrow and uva ursi are both used to combat urinary infections, although you should discontinue the use of uva ursi if the infection continues more than one week. Use liberal amounts of raw garlic or garlic capsules. Rose hip tea and lemon water in large amounts are said to help. Be sure to wipe from front to back after using the bathroom, and to urinate after intercourse, as the germ can spread from the intestines or from your partner. If the infection doesn't clear within a few days, you need to see a doctor.

YEAST INFECTIONS

To treat vaginal infections, such as yeast infections, the same advice goes for sanitary measures. Wear all-cotton underwear, or go without underwear. Don't use tight pants or synthetics near the genitals. Watch your intake of sweets. Take plenty of lemon water or rose hip tea to increase the C-complex intake. Take green drink several times a day, and take apple-cider vinegar in water twice a day to increase the body's acidity. You can douche with a vinegar-water solution, with yogurt, or with an acidophilus solution, but we are very wary of douching during pregnancy. If you live in an area where you can buy homeopathic preparations, the homeopathic candida albicans can work remarkably fast to clear up yeast infections. You should consult a natural practitioner about it. Reduce stress, rest more, and you should clear up the "itch" soon enough with the above remedies.

TOXEMIA

A woman who has followed the mucusless diet throughout her pregnancy, and who has followed the simple herbal program, should not get anywhere near suffering toxemia. The symptoms are water retention, hypertension, and protein in the urine. If you have followed a less-than-ideal program, and are beginning to have toxemia symptoms, try the following suggestions. However, if you don't see immediate progress, see a physician: toxemia is life-threatening. Be sure that you are eating high-quality, adequate protein. Don't limit your intake of salt, but be sure that the salt is from the sea or mineral deposits; however, most sodium needs are easily obtained from fresh greens, especially fresh celery juice. Refined salt is equivalent to refined sugar. The Hunzas, once the prime example of healthy people, began to decline in health when they stopped mining their own coarse salt and began to buy or trade for refined salt. Double your intake of the comfrey-raspberry-alfalfa combination, in green drink if at all possible. Motherwort tea will eliminate the swelling (it is also good for nervousness and depression). Make sure your diet is low stress, including lots of fruits and vegetables, nuts and seeds, with some yogurt or natural cottage cheese. You need more calcium during this time, but don't take calcium pills, because out of proportion, calcium pills aggravate problems in your body. You need approximately twice the amount of phosphorus and a proportion of silica in order to utilize calcium effectively. Take Dr. Christopher's calcium formula and calcium-rich foods, especially greens. Calcium tablets just release free radical calcium into the system and can cause more damage than help. Drink lemon juice and honey or maple syrup throughout the day, as well as plenty of fluids. Get lots of rest and reduce your stress. Increase your potassium intake (bananas, mint, and dandelions are good sources of potassium; dulse and kelp are some of the best sources). Raw beets can help with the potassium in the system. We like to grate beets, combine with chopped celery and grated carrot, and dress with homemade mayonnaise; raw garlic is good in this salad, and it is healing and cleansing. Watch toxemia carefully, in conjunction with your midwife or doctor. It can cause liver damage and death.

HIGH BLOOD PRESSURE

High blood pressure, as ascertained by your practitioner, can be treated herbally. You should not be suffering it if you are following the recommended diet. You can increase your intake of raspberry leaf tea to lower the blood pressure. Garlic and hawthorn berry are proven tonics for this condition, and neither will hurt you or the baby. Exercise and peace of mind can lower blood pressure dramatically. If you are undergoing stress, you need to find a lifestyle solution that will allow you to stop it. Some nutritionists say that raw cucumber, either juiced or in salad, is good for reducing blood pressure! Cayenne is good for this condition. Dr. Christopher's blood pressure formula (B.P.) can lower blood pressure if it's high or raise it if it's low.

HORMONES

Recurring miscarriages can indicate a hormone imbalance, but hormone adjustments are common in pregnancy. As my husband often says, "Your hormones are raging!" A local midwife explained that the estrogen level in a woman is higher at conception, and then the progesterone level goes higher to maintain the pregnancy. When birth is near, the estrogen level rises again until the baby is born. When the ovaries do not produce enough progesterone and the estrogen level remains too high, the mother may lose the baby. Ginseng and/or sarsaparilla contain hormone precursors and can help the body produce progesterone and keep the baby. One capsule a day of sarsaparilla (or a mixture of both) should be enough. Keep up your protein and B-vitamin foods intake to keep your hormone level up. Foods high in hormones include carrots, soybeans, wheat, oats, barley, potatoes, apples, cherries, plums, garlic and rice bran. You should eliminate unnecessary stresses such as community, family, or church commitments for the first three or four months of pregnancy if you are prone to this problem. You can bring up the estrogen level, if you are trying to conceive, by taking 1 or 2 capsules of black cohosh, licorice, blessed thistle or any other female hormone herbs. You can use Dr. Christopher's false unicorn and lobelia formula, and his hormone balancing formula (Changease) which has both the estrogen and progesterone type hormone precursors. When you use herbs which contain these precursors, your body is allowed to select and convert into hormones the precursors that it needs to correct any imbalance. This is so unlike allopathic medicine which gives the actual hormones, not allowing the body to be selective.

MISCARRIAGE

If you are prone to miscarriage, Dr. Christopher recommended a sure course to overcome miscarriages. Early one morning, Dr. Christopher was working in his study, when the telephone rang. It was a lady on one end of Evanston, where he was practicing, asking "Will you come quickly? I am hemorrhaging! I have lost several babies before, and I don't want to lose this one." Dr. Christopher told her to stay in bed, using a bedpan if necessary. She was to have someone prepare hot water. He packed his bag and headed for the door; the phone rang again. This was a lady on the other side of Evanston, asking for him to come quickly, with the same problem! He told her he had another call he had to attend first, but to follow the same instructions. So he repacked his bag with enough herbs for both of them and headed out. He gave them each the same thing, a combination of three parts false unicorn root and one part lobelia, using a teaspoon of the combination to the cup, making a tea and using a half cup every half hour. After the bleeding stopped, they were to take it every hour the rest of the day and then three times a day for the next three days. After he helped the one lady, he went to the other lady and helped her. At the end of the nine months of each pregnancy, each woman had the baby, carried full term, in perfect condition and with no miscarriages.

This combination can also help pass a dead fetus. How does it work in both cases? The lobelia in the formula is a thinking herb. Where the baby is strong, as in the above cases, the lobelia seems to have the knowledge to assist in healing a tearing and bleeding condition and stopping the bleeding. But if the baby is dead and should be aborted, the lobelia has the intelligence of directing the abortion. For example, a lady in American Fork, Utah, became pregnant, but started miscarrying in the fourth or fifth month. Dr. Christopher was out of town, but one of his students came over to give her some help. She brought about five other ladies from the class. They all brought false unicorn with them, but one of them remembered the lobelia. They mixed it together, and gave the woman the tea every half hour. Instead of the bleeding receding and eventually stopping, the bleeding got worse. Five of the ladies got scared and didn't know what to do, because this was new to them, but the sixth lady (the one who brought the lobelia) said, "The doctor said that if the bleeding gets worse, then we have to rush her to the hospital immediately." They called the American Fork Hospital and asked them to prepare a bed for her. They put her in the car and took her to the hospital, which wasn't very far away. When the doctor had her on the table, she started to abort the baby. The doctor gasped, saying, "That baby is dead, and has been dead about six weeks. I have never seen a baby abort itself like this; you must have been using something special." The lady told him she was using an anti-abortion formula. The doctor said, "I'd like to know what it is, but I don't dare, because I would be in trouble if I used it with any of my other patients. But don't forget what this formula is, and remember to use it whenever needed." This formula saved the lady from a stressful D&C, quite a blessing to her.

VITAMINS

Do you need supplements during pregnancy? Most natural practitioners insist that vitamin supplements are necessary to a good pregnancy and delivery, yet you might ask yourself the question, why are vitamins in such minute quantities in food? It is because the body only requires these small amounts. Why then do we insist on taking megadoses of vitamins? It is true that vitamins seem to work, but they eventually weaken the system instead of building it because they continue to assault the body in excessive amounts. There are many foods that can supply rich nutrients if we need extra. For example, many midwives say that vitamin E helps tissues stretch, preventing tearing during a birth. Instead of taking synthetic vitamin E capsules, which do not work for this purpose, many women take natural vitamin E, d-alpha tocopherol; even better would be fresh wheat germ oil, which is rich in the vitamin as well as the natural adjuncts which allow it to work synergistically in the system. We have already discussed iron supplements; the combination of yellow dock and dandelion supplies excellent, assimilable iron. Vitamin C is said to help tissues stretch and to help a woman avoid infections. Instead of taking synthetic C, which lacks the trace elements necessary for effective use, including most importantly the correct proportion of copper, you can take foods rich in C such as citrus, green peppers, rose hips, potatoes-- almost all raw fruits and vegetables. Paprika is extremely rich in vitamin C.

Calcium tablets are almost always prescribed for muscle cramps and throughout pregnancy generally, yet calcium requires the proper balance of phosphorus, silica and magnesium to be absorbed. Otherwise the free-radical calcium flows through the bloodstream, sometimes depositing in the forms of cysts and calcium deposits. Often people who suffer from arthritis and related problems, arteriosclerosis and calcium deposits, are taking plenty of calcium supplements, but their bodies cannot assimilate the calcium in this form. The best calcium supplement you can take, other than calcium-rich foods, is Dr. Christopher's calcium formula formula, which contains exactly the right proportion of silica because of the horsetail grass. Carrot juice is a good source of calcium, and green leafy vegetables contain lots of it. The darker the green, the more calcium it contains. Turnip greens and kale--though not everyone's favorite, it is true--contain several times the calcium contained in milk. If you cream the greens, using a sauce of whole-grain flour, butter and either goat's milk or soy or nut milk, you can serve a mild and calcium-rich dish. Only a few of the B-vitamins have yet been discovered, yet we try to take vitamin pills to supply this need. These vitamins are present in whole grains, brewer's yeast, and seaweeds. Your body will manufacture its own B-vitamins as it needs them if you maintain a proper intestinal flora, which is done by taking sauerkraut, yogurt, acidophilus culture, or rejuvelac (see page 143). Comfrey, dulse, kelp, kale, spinach, soy and other beans, peas and sprouts are some of the vegetable sources of vitamin B-12, an element often claimed lacking in vegetarian diets. Sesame butter is an excellent source of protein and calcium.

We also recommend two other products that should be available in your local health food store or at The Herb Shop, PO Box 777 Springville, UT 84663. These are "Vitalherbs" and "Jurassic Green". Vitalherbs is a combination of herbs formulated to provide whole food quantities of vitamins and minerals in a balance that only nature can provide. Jurassic Green is a blend of alfalfa, wheat grass and barley grass grown organically in a mineral rich, ancient sea bed.

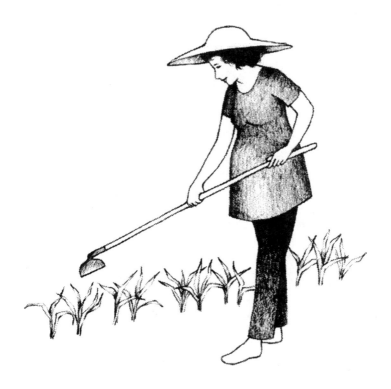

CLEANSING DURING PREGNANCY

Sometimes women during pregnancy and nursing feel that they want to do the three-day cleanse, a fast, or other cleansing procedures. If a woman has regularly been doing the three-day cleanse, it should cause no harm to continue doing this once a month or so. We strongly discourage fasting of any other kind during these periods. If a woman has not already been in the practice of the three-day cleanse, she should not begin during pregnancy or nursing, at least when the baby is taking all of its nourishment from her. A mother desiring to cleanse can be sure that the bowels are kept open, as described on page 37. She can concentrate on cleansing types of foods, such as fruits, raw vegetables, sea vegetables. She can drink plenty of pure water, and take lots of juices. Exercise in the fresh air can cleanse the body. But be patient, and wait to do more direct cleansing until your baby is weaned.

RH FACTOR

Dr. Christopher worked during pregnancies to heal women with serious problems, and his results seem to us miraculous. One of his students from northern Utah had three children with the Rh problem; in each case, they had to have a complete blood transfusion, having their blood completely drained out of them. This lady was told that because of her advanced Rh problem, she was not to have any more children. In addition to the Rh problem, she would require open heart surgery, and another pregnancy might kill not only her, but the child. She asked Dr. Christopher for help. He could promise her nothing, but tried to help her cleanse her blood. She took the red clover combination tea in order to cleanse the blood, the female corrective formula and hormone-balancing formula, and plenty of red raspberry leaf tea. After a lecture some time later, the lady approached Dr. Christopher with a new baby, born naturally with no Rh problem whatsoever. The lady had several children since that time, with no more trouble. This shows that the Rh factor stems from a problem of toxicity inside the mother, which can be overcome with herbs and diet.

VAGINAL BIRTH AFTER CAESAREAN

A lady in Springville, Utah, came to Dr. Christopher's office in Evanston, Wyoming. She had had three children, and her doctor told her the only way she could bear children was by Caesarean section, because she had a pelvic area that was rather immature. She had so much scar tissue on the abdominal area that the doctors said she could not be cut again. She wanted another baby very much so she came to Dr. Christopher to see what he might be able to do. He put her on the three-day cleanse and mucusless diet. She was to drink at least a quart of red raspberry leaf tea a day, to drink a gallon of steam-distilled water a day, and to use the three-oil massage over the abdominal area. That would be two days of castor oil massaging the area, two days of olive oil, and two days of wheat germ oil, and a day of rest. Dr. Christopher felt that if she would follow this program, she would heal rapidly. She also was to take the female corrective formula and the hormone balancing formulas internally, and to keep her bowels clean with the lower bowel formula. She visited Dr. Christopher every week, and began to feel much better. The hardness of her abdomen had softened so that it became pliable. The scar tissue began to show signs of new life.

During this time, Dr. Christopher moved into his offices in Salt Lake City, Utah. Dr. Loretta Foote, who took care of all the obstetric cases, came in one day and said she would be gone for a couple of days, because she was going to assist a lady in delivery down in Springville, a patient of Christopher's. She reminded him of the lady who had had three Caesarean births, who was planning a home delivery. Dr. Foote returned to help the mother for about ten days (in those days it must have been easier than today!). The woman who was told that she could only have C-sections now had natural childbirths at home with ease. Many years later, this lady came up after the lecture, and trailing her were four teenage children; she informed Dr. Christopher that all four of these were born after she'd been told she'd lose her life and her baby's if she dared another birth. She was a very happy woman.

If you faithfully follow the natural program outlined here, you should have a smooth pregnancy and no serious problems. But what if you suspect something is wrong? I believe that a mother's intuition should be trusted, and if you feel a need to see a medical practitioner, by all means follow your womanly wisdom and do so. I tend to consult my lay midwife before I go to the doctor. Yet the medical profession is capable of treating emergencies, and you should feel free to consult a doctor if you feel the need. Otherwise, I feel that the prenatal care supplied by the midwives was superior to that I received from medical doctors. The midwives routinely checked my urine and blood pressure, weight, and fundal height, but did not take blood. I appreciated this, because I do not believe in violating the body's natural barrier, the skin. Most importantly, they spent time answering my questions and observing me generally. Such time-consuming examinations can reveal problems that test-tube testing cannot always do.

BIRTH

A discussion of birth attendants always leads to the important question: Where do I want to give birth? Nowadays there are more options for the pregnant couple than ever before. Hospitals are providing home-like rooms with quilts, rocking chairs and brass beds, including the option of having children and other family members at the birth and visiting afterward. Birthing centers are offering most of these same options, allowing the healthy mother and infant to go home very soon when all is well. Nurse-midwives replace the male presence of the doctor; some doctors admit that women, in the vulnerability and need of the birth process, look to them for the comfort and even love that the father of the baby should supply. However, with all of these options, some drawbacks still exist. Birth in hospitals or like institutions can be fraught with experiences that home births completely avoid. What are the issues in hospital versus home birth?

Clearly, the main advantage of a hospital birth offers emergency care in case of complications. Many women who have suffered unforeseen problems swear by the hospital--they would have lost their baby, they say, if they had been at home. While it is true that hospitals offer incomparable emergency care, statistics show that over 95% of all births proceed normally. Most times, birth problems can be predicted by careful prenatal examination, including careful analysis of a mother's history.

HIGH RISK FOR HOME BIRTH

Some circumstances create questions about the feasibility of a home birth, although they do not necessarily preclude it. Some of these include a previous history of neonatal death; you should analyze carefully why a mother produced a stillborn or a baby that died soon after birth. Several women I know have home-birthed beautiful babies after having a tiny one die in previous circumstances, so this does not preclude home birth, but you should analyze the causes. In particular, diabetes or border-line diabetes, which can threaten a newborn, should be treated herbally.

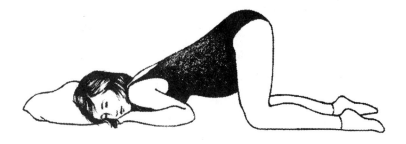

If a woman has a history of repeated malpositioning of the baby, home birth is still possible, but I consider it paramount that the position be carefully checked during the last of the pregnancy. If the baby is malpositioned, some women assume a knee-chest position, resting their head on a pillow and elevating their hips from the knees. This has been said to turn a posterior baby. By lying on your back with a pillow beneath the small of your back twice a day for ten minutes, you can sometimes turn a breech baby; relaxing on a slant board is said to do the same thing. Certainly a prayer and blessing from the father can help with malpositioning. One young woman, bearing her eighth child, felt that it really wasn't in position yet, although the birth time was near. Medical checks indicated that the baby's head was lodged somewhat to the side of the cervix, unable to move. The father blessed the mother that she would experience a normal birth, and the baby's head moved over and engaged correctly. We believe that faith has a good deal to do with a happy birth experience.

The Rh-negative problem doesn't mean you can't give birth at home; you should carefully concentrate on a good diet and herbs, as we indicated in the previous chapter, and monitor the condition of the blood. Usually the problem arises in the third or later pregnancies of an affected mother. If the danger is still present when birth is imminent, carefully discuss the problem with your midwife, and if you and she cannot decide for sure, go to a doctor to determine the exact nature of the condition. In a serious situation, you will have to be delivered in a hospital so that the baby can have a complete blood transfusion. Otherwise, the midwife should be able to take blood from the umbilical cord before it is cut, have it analyzed, and make a decision based on that information. Watch for jaundice in the first two days; this can be a sign of Rh problem; don't be afraid to consult a doctor if you are not sure!

If a mother is extremely overweight, she should seriously analyze her motives and ability to give birth at home. You should not plan to lose weight during a pregnancy, yet obesity makes a labor harder, may cause prematurity, and could cause toxemia and a too-large baby. A good exercise program and superior nutrition are in any case absolutely essential.

If a mother has had a previous abortion, has taken birth control pills, has an IUD left in place or has suffered an incompetent D&C, she should be very careful about deciding on home birth. She could experience complications that such interventions cause, including uterine damage from the abortion and other mechanical interventions, and circulatory problems caused by the birth control pill. The Pill also increases the possibility of blood clots, heart attacks, liver tumors, headaches, depression, and cancer. If a mother has had a suitably long lapse of time after taking the Pill, or if she has taken it for only a short time, there may be no threat to her or her baby.

Any prospective mother who takes drugs, drinks, or smokes should stop totally before pregnancy. If she cannot, she should not accept the responsibility for a home birth. It usually takes about a year to cleanse the body of the ill effects of these materials, although the pregnancy will have to be closely monitored.

On the high risk list for home births would include the following: untreated heart disease, kidney disease, diabetes (extremely dangerous), gestational diabetes (this is where the mother never experienced diabetes before, but pregnancy brings it on), lung disease, cancer, severe asthma or allergies, epilepsy, uncontrolled toxemia, and emotional illness. If you have any of these, morally you are obligated to discuss them fully with a prospective midwife so that she can decide the best course for you. A monitored hospital birth in these circumstances would be better than a tragedy at home.

Quite apart from these ominous warnings, however, reassure yourself that statistics show over 95% of all births to be normal. Most times, complications can be predicted by careful prenatal examination. And in a normal birth, hospital procedures can actually endanger the mother or infant where at home no danger would exist. The few studies that compare statistics of hospital and home births indicate that home birth is indeed safe, and often safer than corresponding births in hospitals. At The Farm, a community that supplies lay midwives for home births, including thorough prenatal care, the average of prenatal deaths was 19.0 per thousand, as compared with nearly double that amount in various hospitals throughout the country. This includes high-risk deliveries that were transported to the hospital; most hospitals do not include in their statistics births transferred to another institution. But by far the most convincing study comparing home birth to hospital birth was done by Lewis Mehl in 1977. Here is an extract of his findings:

PROCEDURE	IN THE HOSPITAL
CAESAREAN OPERATION	Three times greater.
FORCEPS	Twenty times more used.
OXYTOCIN (to accelerate or induce labor)	Twice as much used.
ANALGESIA AND ANESTHESIA	Nine times more used.
EPISIOTOMY	Nine times greater incidence of an episiotomy, while at the same time they had more severe tears in need of major repair in the hospital.
INFANT DISTRESS IN LABOR	Six times more.
MATERNAL HIGH BLOOD PRESSURE	Five times more cases.
POSTPARTUM HEMORRHAGE	Three times greater.

PROCEDURE	IN THE HOSPITAL
INFECTION OF NEWBORN	Four times more infection among the newborn.
BABIES NEEDING HELP TO BREATHE	Three times more babies needed help to begin to breathe.
BIRTH INJURIES	There were THIRTY cases of birth injuries, including skull fractures, facial nerve palsies, brachial nerve injuries and severe cephalhematomas. THERE WERE NO SUCH INJURIES AT HOME.
INFANT DEATH RATE	Infant death rate was low in both cases and essentially the same.
MATERNAL DEATH RATE	There were no maternal deaths for either home or hospital.

His research concluded, in comparing the home births in his area with hospital births throughout California in the year studies.

1973		HOME BIRTH RATE	ALL CALIFORNIA BIRTH RATE
Total Births	1152		
Live Births	1147		
Fetal Death	5	4.3/1000	10.2/1000
Neonatal Deaths	6	5.2/1000	10.3/1000
Total Prenatal Deaths	11	9.5/1000	20.3/1000
Low Birth Weight (2501 g.)	15	1.3%	6.4%

(Mehl, Lewis, et al., "Outcome of Elective Home Birth: A Series of 1147 Cases," *The Journal of Reproductive Medicine,* Vol. 19, No. 5, Nov. 1977, pp. 288-289.) A more detailed breakdown of Mehl's findings can be found in Steward, David and Lee, *Safe Alternatives in Childbirth*, Chapel Hill, NC, NAPSAC, 1976, pp. 73-100. This should be required reading for anyone trying to convince recalcitrant family members to accept their planned home birth.

Birthing at home should be chosen primarily for the safety and happiness of the newborn and mother--not for financial reasons, not for striking out against society, not to spite someone opposing the family's way of life. Most couples undertaking home birth take upon themselves the responsibility for the good outcome of the birth, not placing this stewardship upon the doctor or the hospital. Of primary importance--physically--is the cleanliness of the home environment. Most couples clean their homes thoroughly before giving birth, thus providing a much safer environment for birthing than in hospitals, which are admittedly pathogenic environments. Although things may look clean, linen, equipment, and utensils may often be far from clean. Consider the physician's stethoscope that travels from bare chest to bare chest without being cleansed. Newborn nurseries can be a place to exchange dangerous germs, especially strep and staph. Studies performed on solutions used to cleanse wounds reported that most of them were polluted with some kind of pathogens. During a hospital stay--a rarity in our family--I watched attendants cleaning carpets, floors and utensils. They did an adequate job, but not the kind I would like during birth or illness in my own home. Technicians handling equipment seemed not to care about washing hands between rooms, and so on.

But of even more importance, during labor and delivery the mother can completely avoid unwanted drugs and use of forceps, both of which offer real problems from the neonate. Most doctors readily admit that there is no drug which is truly safe for the baby. Many mothers lament their sluggish, unresponsive, ever-sleepy babies after a drugged birth. A recent study showed that babies born to mothers given anesthetics during delivery were much more apt to suffer physical and mental impairment. These drugs included Demerol and Seconal, considered mild and given to relax the mother in early labor, anesthetics which are inhaled, such as nitrous oxide, and injected anesthetics of the Procaine family (*The People's Doctor*, Vol. 3, No. 3, p. 2). Mothers report headaches and back troubles for years after undergoing anesthesia in childbirth. And too often, forceps delivery, which can bruise the baby and traumatize a very tender young head, will follow anesthesia, as the mother is not able to feel the pushing contractions and cannot deliver the baby herself. Most mothers are offered anesthesia as they go into transition, when emotions are most vulnerable and the mother least resistant; the most common comment during transition seems to be, "I just can't do this any more." This is a sign that birth is not long away, that the mother is dilated almost fully. To offer a woman anesthesia at this point is cruel, especially since the pushing stage of birth is not usually painful, but rather very satisfying, and the birthing moment itself may offer little pain as well. Without anesthesia, mothers and babies remain alert and the birthing process goes normally and usually faster.

Home birth also avoids the use of ultrasound during labor, which is what fetal monitors are--prolonged exposure to ultrasound waves. External monitors have proven to be somewhat inaccurate, especially if the mother moves (and who wants to remain stationary during labor; who can stay still during labor?) Several reports have shown that babies who have been monitored have died during labor, although the machine hadn't shown any problem to warn the doctors (*The People's Doctor*, Vol. 3, No. 3, p.5). Internal fetal monitoring, which often requires breaking of the waters before necessary, which increases needlessly the intensity of the contractions and can jam the baby's head repeatedly against the mother's pubic bones, has caused scalp abscess, uterine perforation, and maternal damage. One report describes an infant who died on the seventh day of life of a disseminated herpes simplex infection introduced at the site on the baby's scalp where the monitoring electrode had been screwed in.

Perhaps not so life-threatening but still, to me, of real importance is the issue of internal exams. I had my first baby in the hospital, where I was examined routinely throughout my labor to determine how many centimeters I was dilated. Sometimes a considerate nurse would wait until after a contraction to uncover me, insert her gloved hand, and check my dilation, but most often they would check me when they entered the room. Research indicates that routine internal exams are a major cause of premature rupture of the membranes. This subjects mother and fetus to the risk of both illness and death from infection. The routine internal examinations open up a pathway for bacteria to enter the cervix and produce infection and ruptured membranes. In this study, the incidence of Caesarean sections was more than twice as high in women whose membranes were ruptured prematurely than in those whose membranes remained intact (*The People's Doctor*, Vol. 8, No. 10, p. 4).

It is not necessary to check a mother's dilation routinely, unless there seems to be a problem with slow labor or other indication, which midwives or doctors can identify. There is a sure indicator that birth is approaching--transition and the urge to push. At that time the birth attendant can check for full dilation and help the mother follow the appropriate course, either waiting a couple of contractions until dilation is complete, or going ahead and pushing.

For the mother's comfort, home birth can avoid routine enemas and prepping--that is, shaving the pubic area. One irreverent observer considered shaving the pubic area before birth as needful as shaving a man's mustache before a tonsillectomy. A mother can bathe, if her water has not broken, right up until time to push. She can shower, even if her water has broken, perhaps sitting on a chair and letting the hot water relax her. Mothers who have used water therapy during labor say that dilation proceeds very rapidly this way. For three of my nine births, I labored in the bathtub right up until transition. Typically, I feel strongly to get out at some point, which usually turns out to be transition. Many hospitals now offer a hot tub or whirlpool for laboring mothers! Very essential, the mother can eat or drink as she pleases during the labor. Medical practice forbids this, as perhaps the mother will have to undergo a C-section, which surgical procedure precludes food in the system. Most women, however, welcome light food and drink--more about this later--as they labor, to keep their energy levels up. Since my own labors are usually precipitous--which means that they happen hard and fast--I rarely eat anything, but I rely heavily on the midwives shock formula, which is a cup of warm water with 2 tablespoons apple cider vinegar, an eighth cup honey, and a full teaspoonful of cayenne. This stops the onset of shock, which I seem to experience with every labor, as well as warming the body, increasing circulation, raising the blood sugar to provide energy, and preventing hemorrhage danger.

Perhaps the most comforting aspect of home birth is that you can stay home! How well I remember the onset of my first labor. First thing in the morning--with a sneeze--my water broke, and we began preparing to go to the hospital. Although the labor was quite mild, since it was my first child I concentrated on the sensations and felt quite a bit of discomfort. My water was gushing out all over the place, and my first placement of a sanitary napkin soon proved to be simply humorous. We gathered my few belongings and, cushioned on a pile of towels, off I went to the hospital. My husband walked me into the receiving area, and I had to ride in a wheelchair up an elevator into a labor room, where I underwent the usual enema, prep and undressing before I was deposited on a labor bed in a drab, small labor room.

What a contrast to my other births, which all took place in my own home, which we had invariably turned upside down and scrubbed a week or more before birth. When the water broke or when contractions became strong, I simple called the appropriate people and went to my own bed. It is so comfortable to approach birth in this way--no getting in and out of cars, no entering a strange place and being subjected to unfamiliar and unwanted routines.

Long before home birth became as accepted as it is today, Dr. Christopher was advocating it; he and his wife had all five of their children at home. A very dramatic example: One lady came to Dr. Christopher's office in Orem with a severe case of cancer. Parts of her body had been cut out; she had lost one arm--her right arm, which was particularly sad because she was an artist. However, she decided that she was going to fight the cancer naturally, and came to Christopher's to learn to be an herbalist. She planned to learn to use her left hand for her art, and she learned iridology and reflexology. She did some art work for Dr. Christopher's charts and books, and was learning to use her left hand very well. But the doctors had told her that she should never get pregnant, because there was cancer all through her body, which would kill both her and the baby. One day, however, she decided that she wanted another baby; she already had three or four children, but she wanted another. She had been in the cleansing program and mucusless diet for some time, and had become stronger. She conceived, the baby developed, and the herb class watched her with admiration. One day in class, a bad snowstorm came up, and through the swirling snow came this lady. She said that she had to come this morning and show them what she had. She threw back her shawl, showing one of the most beautiful babies Dr. Christopher had seen. She had birthed it the night before. She had delivered the baby herself, with one hand, and didn't bother her husband, although when it came time to tie and cut the cord, she had to wake him for help. Dr. Christopher considered this most unusual, for a woman who had had cancer and suffered all the operations that she had, and yet here she had delivered her own baby at home.

Other advantages of home birth include your own choice of birthing position, and, most frequently, the paramount advantages for the newborn; she can lie quietly on the mother's abdomen until the cord stops pulsating completely, thus easing gently into the new business of breathing. The baby rests warm in the mother's arms; if there is vernix left on the skin, much of it may remain and help nourish the skin; the baby can nurse immediately.

Is home birth an underground, fringy sort of thing? Resoundingly no! More and more women are undertaking home birth, largely from the natural lifestyle movement, but sometimes not. Some--but not many--medical doctors are advocating the safety of home birth. And the legal issues of home birth are being addressed more and more.

MIDWIFERY AND LAW

Of course, the legality of home birth is significantly a moral question. Mothers and fathers should be able to choose their birth place anywhere they desire. Unfortunately the laws in some states sometimes consider the practice of lay midwifery medical practice, and midwives have endured some difficulties. In Utah, although there have been some attempts to curb the practice of lay midwifery, it is not considered the practice of medicine, and parents are legally given the right to deliver their baby where, when, and how and with whom they choose regardless of certification (Senate Bill #243, 8 May 1979). In Alaska, naturopathic physicians and midwives who were delivering, especially in outlying areas, were legally accosted and asked to cease and desist their practice. After an intense and wearying struggle, The Midwives Association of Alaska lobbied and won the legal right to practice. Before employing a lay midwife, check with your state law to see whether midwifery is considered the practice of medicine. The following gives an idea of the current status of state laws on midwifery.

ALABAMA   Legal only for "granny" midwives, but some others
                do practice covertly.

ALASKA   Now legal. More regulation is expected.

ARIZONA   Legal if licensed, but lay midwives do practice
                covertly.

ARKANSAS   Legal if licensed, though licenses are restricted, but lay midwives practice anyway.

CALIFORNIA   Illegal, but lay midwives do practice, sometimes with harassment. New legislation pending.

COLORADO   Illegal, but lay midwives practice and are sometimes harassed. New legislation pending.

CONNECTICUT   Legislation exists only for certified nurse midwives. No regulation for lay midwives, however good relations exist.

DELAWARE   Permits available only to midwives from the American College of Nurse Midwives. A few lay midwives practice covertly.

DISTRICT OF COLUMBIA   Illegal, difficult to find a lay midwife.

FLORIDA   Difficult to obtain yet legal if licensed. Lay midwives practice covertly.

GEORGIA   Unclear legal status. No certification available even though its required by law. Lay midwives practice, usually covertly.

HAWAII   Only certified nurse midwives can attend home birth legally. Some lay midwives practice covertly.

IDAHO   Legal because of lack of legislation; lay midwives practice.

ILLINOIS   Illegal since 1963, but lay midwives continue. New legislation pending.

INDIANA   Illegal, but active home birth movement with lay midwives. Only Certified Nurse midwives are licensed.

IOWA   No specific law. A 1978 attorney general's opinion

concluded that midwifery is practicing medicine without a license. Lay midwives practice discreetly.

KANSAS No legislation, and lay midwives practice.

KENTUCKY Legal if licensed (which is currently impossible to obtain). Lay midwives practice in the open.

LOUISIANA A licensing procedure for midwives was finalized in June 1988. Licensed midwives practice openly. "Granny" midwives practice covertly.

MAINE No legislation, and lay midwives practice. Attorney general's opinion records that midwifery is not the practice of medicine.

MARYLAND Illegal, and lay midwives difficult or impossible to find. Licensure restricted to Certified Nurse Midwives.

MASSACHUSETTS Lay midwives practice openly. State Supreme Court decision of 1985 makes it illegal for nurses to practice midwifery. No regulation exists to prohibit lay persons from practicing.

MICHIGAN Legal, and midwives available.

MINNESOTA Laws ambiguous, but midwives actively practice. By definition only gratuitous emergency service is legal.

MISSISSIPPI Legal according to law but attitudes are poor. Lay midwives keep a low profile and fear harassment.

MISSOURI Presently illegal except for trained RN's. A few lay midwives continue to practice. Positive legislation is being actively sought.

MONTANA Legal as of April 11, 1989. Midwives practice openly.

NEBRASKA Laws ambiguous, but emotional climate unfavorable. Some midwives do practice.

NEVADA Laws ambiguous, legislative climate favorable while physicians actively against. Some midwives practice openly.

NEW HAMPSHIRE Bill establishing the option to certify as a lay midwife was passed July 1981. Lay midwives practice openly.

NEW JERSEY Illegal, midwives limited and practice quietly. Only Certified Nurse Midwives are granted licenses.

NEW MEXICO Legal with very favorable climate and thriving open practice.

NEW YORK Illegal, but many lay midwives practice openly.

NORTH CAROLINA Illegal, although some do practice. Large community support.

NORTH DAKOTA Legal, with an improving emotional climate. Very few lay midwives practice.

OHIO Stringent certification process inhibits legal practice. Several lay midwives practice openly.

OKLAHOMA Midwifery is not legally defined or prohibited. Lay midwives practice openly.

OREGON Positive legislative status with support form attorney general's opinion. Midwives practice openly and are politically active.

PENNSYLVANIA Illegal, but some lay midwives practice openly where community support is strong.

RHODE ISLAND Legal with license (which is difficult to obtain).

A few unlicensed midwives practice covertly.
Medical community is hostile.

SOUTH CAROLINA   Legal with registration. Positive legislative and community support.

SOUTH DAKOTA   Not legally defined and not prohibited. As of 1990 no lay midwives could be found.

TENNESSEE   Legal with active and thriving lay midwifery practice.

TEXAS   Legal and very active home birth movement with lay midwives.

UTAH   Legal with active lay midwifery movement.

VERMONT   Legal and midwives practice.

VIRGINIA   Illegal without permit which is not available to new applicants. Lay midwives practice with community support.

WASHINGTON   Legal with license. Licensure is available and provides a large degree of freedom to practice. Lay midwives also practice openly without license.

WEST VIRGINIA   Illegal, but still some lay midwives practice. Health Department is currently exploring the possibility of a training program for lay midwives.

WISCONSIN   Ambiguous, Nurse midwifery was legalized in 1980. Lay midwives do practice.

WYOMING   Legal, but emotional climate hostile. By interpretation, midwives can attend home births but they cannot give prenatal or post natal care. Some lay midwives practice openly.

(For a more detailed report on state law, contact *Mothering Magazine*, PO Box 1690, Santa Fe, NM 87504)

Of course there are other considerations to choosing a midwife. The InterNational Association of Parents and Professionals for Safe Alternatives in Childbirth (NAPSAC), Route 1, Box 646 Marble Hill, MO 63764, (314) 214-2010 can sometimes be of help in directing you to midwifery help in your area. You may be surprised to find listings in the yellow pages under birth, midwifery, etc. Usually health food stores or cooperatives, or perhaps naturopaths, chiropractors or other naturally-oriented practitioners can point you in the right direction. Once you have a list of midwives, don't just blindly choose one and hope for the best. Talk to other women who have employed them. But most importantly, sit down with the midwife for a chat, perhaps at a meal. If you feel any unease or distressing feelings, listen to yourself closely. Make it a matter of prayer and meditation. Choose carefully and slowly. You may not always understand the reasons for the intuitive messages you are getting, but trust them. Our experience has shown that you can be led to just the right midwife or practitioner for your emotional and spiritual needs, in addition to your physical needs.

When the time of birth is approaching, most women feel miserably huge and anxious to get on with the birth. Sometimes they act upon these feelings by trying to get birth started. If you are taking the prenatal herbal formula, this in itself should be preparing the muscles and responses necessary to start birth on time. If you really think you are going over your due date, you might try taking some blue cohosh in capsules, tea, or tincture form. Blue cohosh will increase contractions if the birth time is right, but if it's not time yet, the contractions will stop.

Some women use castor oil to induce labor; I have tried this, and it does start some contractions, but they stop if it is not time to give birth. However, if a mother has problems during pregnancy, castor oil could possibly cause premature birth, so I wouldn't use it if there were any question. Castor oil is mixed with orange juice and baking soda by some; some mix it with vodka and orange juice. Some just take it straight.

You could rub castor oil on your belly, which seems to be a safer approach. Some people take a tea made of dried parsley. Some take labor tinctures, as for example 3 parts lady slipper root, 2 parts wild yam, 1 part ginger root, made into tincture or tea. Some increase their dosage of the prenatal formula if they think they are overdue.

Personally, I have come to believe that in most cases the baby's spirit initiates the changes that bring on birth. Of course, there are always cases of babies being overdue, and you and your midwife or doctor will be able to ascertain if you are one of them. Most of the time, in healthy pregnancy, I would take my prenatal formula, raspberry tea, and green drink, continue my healthy diet, go for weeks, and wait for the day. Each baby has its own birth day, the day it is meant to be born. Each baby is born in its own way. Even though we become tired and impatient (and I think it's meant to be that way), we need to grow from the experience of waiting. Each time I am ready to give birth, I tell myself that I will be calm and accepting of the baby's proper birth day. Rarely do I accomplish it! But I am learning the process of waiting for everything in its season, its proper time.

ONSET OF LABOR

How can you tell if you're in labor? Especially if you're expecting your first child, labor may seem a long time in coming and then a long time in process! Active labor follows no preset pattern, although the medical profession has set some standards: If the contractions increase in duration and decrease in time between, you can usually call it true labor. But many women have irregular contractions and are still progressing rapidly. Some labors begin with a bloody show, which is bloody-tinged mucus. If the water breaks, labor usually begins, but sometimes if this happens labor doesn't start for some time after. If you experience this, be in constant contact with your midwife or doctor. A study by Lewis Mehl showed that you can go for about four days after premature rupture of the membranes without an increased risk of infection, but we suggest you do not subject yourself to unnecessary risk. Certainly if you start even a mild fever, seek immediate medical help. If you decide to watch and wait, be sure to keep yourself fastidiously clean. You can take garlic and echinacea to reduce the risk of infection. Be sure to wipe yourself from front to back. Some midwives encourage the use of toilet paper that has been "baked" in a 200 degree F. oven for an hour to eliminate bacteria. One young mother's water broke, but labor didn't start for almost two days. Contractions began on their own, however, and the baby was born, healthy and strong, although the descent through the "dry" birth canal was painful.

You can usually be sure if you're in labor if your contractions make it difficult to do anything else. If your water hasn't broken, you can take a good, hot bath if you suspect you're in labor. True labor will continue while false labor will subside. If you suspect you're in labor, scrub and disinfect the tub before bathing.

PREPARATORY LABOR

Don't suppose that contractions that stop are doing no good, however. I don't believe in the term "false labor." I usually call it preliminary labor, as the many contractions I experience preceding birth--sometimes up to two months before birth--thin the cervix and begin dilation. During my later pregnancies, I have often "started" labor dilated to four or five centimeters. The water breaking initiates a series of good contractions that send me almost immediately into transition, and my babies are often born an hour or so after supposedly true labor starts.

SELF-EXAM

If your water hasn't broken, you can examine yourself internally to see how you're doing, provided you are careful and clean about it. In a tub of comfortably hot water, recline and, with soap-scrubbed hands, insert your longest finger in to reach the cervix. An undilated cervix feels like a rubber tip on a balloon, or like the tip of your nose. The cervix will begin to soften and thin out, until it feels like your tongue or a soft, warm balloon full of water. If you are dilating, you can feel the opening; a "smiley" or semi-circular opening means you are making progress but not in serious labor yet. A round opening can mean that labor is not far away. And if you feel a protrusion of your bag of waters, be extremely gentle and look forward to your labor, because it's near!

Some women experience real discomfort with preliminary labor, a pinching sort of cramping feeling. If you have this problem, soak in a good warm ginger bath. If you feel you are having too many contractions too early, you should take capsules of the false unicorn-lobelia combination, or Siberian ginseng. Both of these should stop premature labor. If there is a serious concern about premature labor, be sure to contact your midwife or doctor.

PRENATAL FORMULA

Five or six weeks before you are due, at about the time you begin to take Dr. Christopher's prenatal formula, you should assemble the materials you will need for the birth. We pack them into a small cardboard box or a clean dishtub, ready to use. You will need the following:

SUPPLIES FOR HOME BIRTH

For the birthing bed, you will need to sterilize a piece of plastic large enough to fit under the mother and surround her. A good wiping with a cloth moist with Clorox water should be adequate; do both sides. Fold it up and wrap it in a paper bag. In very hot water, wash a white cotton sheet in detergent and Clorox. Also wash some washcloths and towels in the same batch. Rinse twice, and dry in a very hot dryer. When the dryer goes off, with soap-scrubbed hands, fold the linen neatly and seal in a paper bag. This bag can be put into a 200 degree F. oven if necessary, if your birth date long passes what you expect. You should also have ready a clean set of bed linen for after the birth. When labor begins, some of us like to make the bed with the clean linen, put the plastic sheet and sterile sheet on top, and remove the soiled things afterwards to a freshly made bed.

You will need some 4x4 sterile gauze pads for supporting the perineum during pushing and for removing any feces that emerge with pushing. You will also need two cord clamps, plastic or metal; or you can buy some new white shoelaces; boil them or soak them in alcohol. This is to tie the cord. (Cord clamps are much easier to use.) You will need some scissors to cut the cord; one blunt point is preferable but not necessary. You will boil these for twenty minutes when labor begins and put them in a bowl, covering them with rubbing alcohol. For each birth, it's ideal to purchase a new bulb syringe, a three-ounce ear syringe. This should be boiled for twenty minutes, and stored in a plastic bag after it is cool. This syringe suctions mucous out of the nose and mouth of the newborn. If the midwife does not supply them, or if your husband will be doing internal exams, you should buy Betadine solution for scrubbing up, and a package of sterile gloves. Also put away a new, small bottle of pure olive oil for perineal massage, so you can stretch the tissues as the baby crowns.

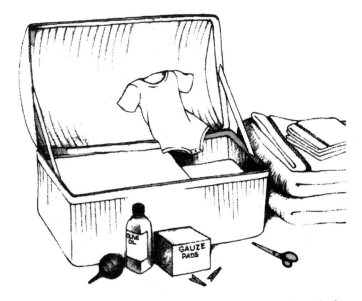

For after the birth, it's best to purchase some underpads from a drug store to place under the mother's hips during the first few days of heavy flow. Buy hospital-sized sanitary napkins and a nice wide belt to hold them. We have made T-binders to wrap around the belly and hold the napkins, but we find the belt easier and cleaner to use. You will need some additional 4x4 gauze squares to cut a hole in the middle and place gently over the cord stump to protect it and keep it clean. Some people swab alcohol on the cord to help it dry up, but we prefer sprinkling it with golden seal powder or myrrh powder; both are antiseptic and healing. Buy at least one package of disposable diapers, newborn size, as the baby's meconium (first bowel movement, very sticky and black) will permanently stain your white cotton diapers. (Pre-made home birth kits can be purchased from The Herb Shop, PO Box 777 Springville, UT 84663)

BABY CLOTHES

You will want to buy clothes for the baby. Follow Dr. Christopher's advice and use no synthetics on the baby (or yourself). You will need undershirts and nighties, perhaps some kimonos and some booties. Get about a half dozen receiving blankets, to swaddle the baby. Most infants really desire this close wrapping. If you have never seen receiving blankets in use, try to visit a family with a newborn, or ask your midwife. For my first baby, I did not even know what receiving blankets were used for! Use all-cotton diapers after the meconium has stopped; you can use plastic pants or, if you can afford them, the lovely diaper covers in natural-fiber catalogs. Don't forget to buy diaper pins.

LABOR HERBS

Be sure you have in the home all the herbs you wish to use. Tinctures are preferable to teas in labor; only a few drops supply the factors available in a cup of tea. Be sure that you have cayenne, vinegar, and honey for the shock tea. Even if you do not tend to shock, it will warm you up and give you energy. Also put in a supply of good-quality juice, both for during the labor and afterward. We always enjoy a drink of pure grape juice after birth--it's sort of a tradition with us. We have bought grape juice in the past, but none of it compared with my husband's home-canned grape juice. The midwives always enjoy this juice after the birth as well.

Any other equipment should be supplied by the midwife or doctor; if you're in doubt, show him or her what you have and see if they require anything else. I also put in a bottle of Dr. Bach's Rescue Remedy, a homeopathic preparation made of flower essences, notably rock rose. This gives wonderful strength and calm during labor, and also can help a slow infant start to breathe.

Along the same line, there is a Smooth Birthing Formula made, similar to the Bach remedies, which can be taken a month before birth, continuing through labor. Both of these preparations are mild and non-harmful, working on the subtle energies of the body and spirit. I have used them and consider them effective.

Keep your box of birth supplies in your birthing room. Be sure that everything is clean, dust-free, and pleasant, and most especially, uncluttered. Have enough pillows or cushions ready for you to semi-sit when you are ready to push your baby out. You'll need them to support your knees as well. Store a pile of newspapers to cover the carpet from your room to the bathroom, to protect the flooring from amniotic fluid as you go back and forth.

Every labor is so different, each in itself. I believe that the progress of the labor reflects in some way the child who is being born. For example, my second son, Sam, was quiet and docile in the womb. I went into labor with my water breaking and called my husband and our friends who were going to assist (the wife of the couple has become a superior midwife, although this was one of her first births). The contractions became more and more intense, but my assistants said, "Don't push, breathe, don't push." My body wanted to push, but I followed their instructions, and soon I said, "I think it's here." Sure enough, his head was out, and after they removed the cord from around the neck, the rest of him slithered out. This quiet and gentle birth reflected the sensitive nature of my Sam.

On the other hand, my third son's labor began with a big pop at 11:00 at night; water gushed out. My husband turned on the light, went to call the midwife and our friend who would assist preparing herb teas, etc., and came back to me. Meanwhile, I had experienced an extremely intense contraction, one I could not handle. We breathed through three or four more of these very strong contractions, my husband pressing the zones on my hands to relieve the pain, holding me all the while, and the two assistants arrived. I was feeling pushy, and in a couple more contractions, our son Jonathan was born--thirty minutes and seven contractions in all! This same baby walked at eight months, throwing himself off furniture until he found his balance. His personality manifested itself at his birth.

Interestingly, labor began with my water breaking with four of six of my boys, but with my girls, I labored until I was fully dilated, whereupon the midwife broke the water--at my request--and the babies were born. Chava, my first girl, was born after a long, gentle labor; we had only an hour of real work, and she gently emerged. With Sarah, our present baby, I had much preparatory labor, often thinking that I was really in labor, only to find it stopping. By the time I was ready to give birth, I think I must have been halfway dilated. I woke up at about two in the morning to go to the bathroom, and began to feel as though there were hands all around the opening of my cervix, steadily pulling it open. I also felt like I was going into shock. When I told my husband I was in labor, he found it hard to believe because of all the false starts we had been having. I was sure, though, so he called our midwives and my friend who would prepare the teas and take care of the running around. We have always chosen a special friend to do this and to experience the birth with us, and for all of us it has become a sacred and bonding experience.

When Diane, our midwife, heard that I was feeling shocky, she was sure I must be in labor, and so she and her assistant rushed through the snowy night to our home far out in the country. Cathy, her assistant, arrived first, just as I was wanting to push. I asked her to please break the waters, as I was ready to push. She didn't want to do that! Diane had told her not to do any exams because I give birth so fast. So I breathed through a couple more contractions until Diane arrived. She scrubbed up and broke my waters, and I began to push in earnest.

I was lying fairly flat, and the pushing wasn't too effective, so we all decided I should be propped up. Except for a few cramps in the legs as the baby descended I experienced almost no pain at all. This was due partially to the good preparation we had done, including walks and baths, nutrition and herbs, but also to the use of zone therapy.

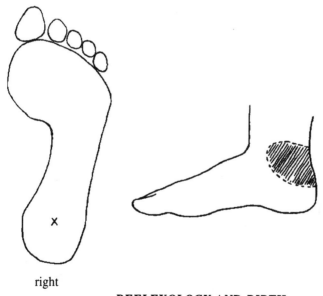

right

REFLEXOLOGY AND BIRTH

During all my home births, I have asked the attendants to press the ankle zones of my feet to help with the pain, the right foot during labor and the left foot to expel the placenta. I had recently read, however, about the use of large combs in the hands to work the zones to relieve pain. You can press the tines of the combs on the fingertips, on the pads just below the fingers, or across the heel of the hands. I always prefer this last position, and would press the combs at the onset of a contraction, putting my hands against my husband, who held me with each contraction and helped me breathe quietly and effectively. I can honestly say that, except for the couple of cramps I felt pushing the baby out, this birth was painless.

What about the moaning and groaning that precede the pushing stage? I used to believe that these were signals of pain, and I tried to suppress them. Reading birth books convinced me that they are a signal that the body is about ready to push. I decided beforehand to let myself groan if I felt like it, and not to be afraid or ashamed of the groans. Sure enough, just as always the sounds came, the characteristic, "Aaah, aaah, and I accepted them for what they were. It was the easiest transition I had ever experienced.

Throughout the labor, I would sip the shock tea, which tastes glorious during labor, as strong as it might seem for other times! We used almost two quarts of it, and when it began to work, my usually cold feet warmed up and I felt glowing all over. (You can wear warm socks for your cold feet too.) The characteristic shaking feeling just disappeared, although usually I shake uncontrollably after the water breaks. Although the cayenne is said to dissipate its hemorrhage stopping effects rather quickly, I never lose much blood at all, and I attribute that at least in part to the shock tea.

Soon the head was crowning, and my husband went in the bathroom to scrub up. He was taking his time--too long--and the head was being born. "You'd better hurry, Avraham, you're going to miss it!" Diane called to him. So he rushed in and felt for the cord around the neck (it wasn't there) and I pushed out a baby girl. He caught her and gently gave her to the midwives, who put her on my abdomen. She lay there, breathing softly, sleeping! After a few moments, she opened her eyes and looked around, as pink and round and soft as can be. We just sat and loved her, feeling the peculiar euphoria that comes with birth--some people say it's like angels all around, and I believe that's true.

After the cord stopped pulsating, the midwives clamped it and Avraham cut it. They took the baby to wash her (they don't remove all of the vernix, but some of it) and weigh her (8-1/2 pounds, my next-to-largest child). My dear friend who came to help with the birth got her dressed in a little cotton rosebud nightgown which I had saved, hoping for a baby girl.

I got out of bed and went for a shower, my husband supporting me along the way. All cleaned up, baby and I got into the newly-made bed and I drank juice while she latched right on and nursed happily.

The midwives kept commenting on the good tone of my tissues and the ease with which I gave birth--and also on the way Avraham and I prepared so well. I believe that we could handle my fast and normal deliveries without assistance, but I love to have the expertise and calm that the lay midwives bring. My third girl, Miriam, was born in fifteen minutes, four contractions, just as you hear in the stories. I have no explanation for this, other than it was a blessing! She's a real blessing, too.

I am saving a brief story of the birth of our fifth child--a son--for a moment, but I believe that these simple stories of natural childbirth are all the more meaningful when you compare them with the practices of birth in hospitals. As one European physician put it, "Since all the physician can really do to affect the course of childbirth for the 95% of mothers who are capable of giving birth without complication is to offer the mother pharmacological relief from discomfort or pain and to perform an episiotomy, there is probably an unconscious tendency for many professionals to see these practices as indispensable" (The Cultural Warping of Childbirth, International Childbirth Education Association). Most women must accept an episiotomy and postpartum shot of oxytocin to prevent hemorrhage and harden the uterus, even if they insist to their doctors that they wish a natural birth. Doctors and nurses routinely offer medication even though the mother has predetermined that she doesn't wish for it; a mother in labor is extremely suggestible, and will often choose drugs in intense labor. This suggestibility can be a very good thing; it makes a mother dependent upon her husband and labor assistants, who can gently encourage her and guide her through the labor with sensitivity and accuracy. Medically-oriented personnel will offer their alternatives to this support, and many women cannot resist it.

Along with the widespread and unneeded use of drugs, unnecessary surgery attends most births. If the husband or midwife gently massages the perineum with olive oil, applies warm compresses, and guides the birthing moment gently, most women can stretch adequately to accommodate the heads and bodies of their babies. Even if some tearing does occur, it is often much less extreme than an episiotomy. I know from experience that a healing episiotomy is extremely uncomfortable; during my other births, I only tore once, with the precipitous Yoni, and that in such a minor way that it only required one or two stitches, given without anesthesia.

Of more serious concern than episiotomies, however, is the growing number of Caesarean sections performed throughout the United States. Twenty years ago, only one baby out of twenty was delivered by C-section, but now the number has risen to one out of four. Doctors may choose to section a woman if the baby is malpositioned, whereas in "old-fashioned" practice, breech or posterior babies were delivered vaginally, sometimes turned in utero by the practitioner. Most doctors insist that a woman who has had a C-section must deliver all her subsequent children in the same way, although many women are questioning this stance, delivering vaginally after their Caesareans, commonly known as VBAC (vaginal birth after Caesarean). *Mothering Magazine* frequently runs inspiring articles by women who have had successful VBAC'S, sometimes at home. They sell a special reprint of an article exploring the issues of Caesarean birth ("Caesarean Special") and occasionally give resources for women to find out more about the issues of VBAC (i.e. Nancy Wainer Cohen, co-founder of C/SEC Inc., 10 Great Plain Terrace, Needham, MA 02192, who offers specialized information on VBAC, including the names of sympathetic practitioners). NAPSAC, P.O. Box 267, Route 1, Box 646 Marble Hill, MO 63734, or the American College of Home Obstetrics, 2821 Rose Street, Franklin Park, IL 60131, both supply names of doctors who support VBAC.

A naturopathic physician told this story at one of Dr. Christopher's lectures. He had had a patient for three pregnancies. Two times she had carried the baby breech, and the doctors had taken them Caesarean. The third time, she happened to be carrying the baby breech, the same pattern as before, and she expected she would have to be operated on again. She began to take Dr. Christopher's pre-natal formula and began to assure herself that the baby would be born normally. Her obstetrician said that it was impossible; no matter how good the formula is, it cannot work. When labor began, the baby was still in the breech position. The obstetrician said to put the lady on the table to prepare to operate, but she said, "No, when it's ready to come, it will turn and come out right." The obstetrician said, "That's ridiculous!" He had put on one rubber glove; the lady screamed, "Here it comes!" Before the obstetrician got the other rubber glove on, the baby came, head first, having previously flipped over. He had to catch it with one hand while the nurse was putting on the other glove. The obstetrician confided to this naturopath that he thought this could never happen. But with the use of the prenatal tea the baby came out normal.

To me, the greatest contrast between my hospital and home births came after the birth. Contrast the gentle handling of my baby girl, Sarah, to what happened to my first son, David. When he was born ("It's a boy!"), they whisked him off while the doctor repaired my episiotomy. I assume they washed, weighed, and dressed him. I was given a clean (warm) gown to wear and the bed cranked up, and David was deposited in my arms for about five minutes. They took him away and wheeled me off to the recovery room, where they brought me supper and we called a few relatives. I was then wheeled to a hospital room with three other women and left to sleep.

During the night, I woke up. "Where is my baby?" I agonized. I sat there in bed, alone, aching, feeling bewildered and confused. The only comfort that helped me through it was a sweet, angelic feeling in the room that assured me that both baby and I were fine. The next morning at 8:00 a.m., a nurse wheeled in a cart full of plastic boxes containing babies. David wasn't the least bit interested in nursing ("too tired, sleepy," they say), but I tried, and held him close. The routine was repeated at noon, but at about 2:00 p.m. we checked out of the hospital and took him home.

Whereupon he began to nurse frantically every two hours, twenty-four hours a day, for nearly a year! When I compare this experience to the early nursing of my other children, who often sucked continuously for hours after the birth, I can only mourn. In our treatment of breastfeeding in the chapter "The New Baby", you will be interested in the research which supports early breastfeeding.

If you run into some problems during labor, certain practices can help you out. If your labor seems slow or sluggish, you might want to assume that you are not really in labor at all. Get up and do the dishes, make a meal, eat, take a walk, have a shower or bath (this only if the water hasn't broken), and go to bed. Don't be anxious. You can envision your cervix opening up, and mentally encourage your contractions. Enjoy a happy talk with your husband and/or birth attendants. If you suspect that you are harboring some fear or tension about birth that is holding things up, you can remind yourself that women have given birth since the beginning of time, and have handled it happily. You can renew your religious faith that God will help you through, and you can reassure yourself that the reflexology techniques (foot massage, hand massage with or without combs, back massage) can help you through the worst moments. You can mentally rehearse the herbs that you will use to cut any unbearable pain.

If you feel that labor should be resumed but is not, you can take blue cohosh, which will bring on good contractions if birth is imminent. You can also make a tea of the prenatal formula which contains herbs that can speed up appropriate labor. Sometimes tincture of lobelia can relax your whole body and your cervix enough to help you open up. A good strong foot massage and perhaps a whole body massage can help resume contractions. Some midwives have located the middle of the heel as the specific place for accupressure to facilitate contractions (see illustration in section on "Reflexology and Birth" on page 71). Midwife and herbalist Margo Bingham suggests a location just to the side of this center place, one a little lower to open a woman up to five centimeters, another a tiny bit higher to open her up the rest of the way. The massage in this case has to be deep and effective, and Margo admits that hardly anyone is able to get it just right, but it's worth a try, especially if it feels good to the laboring woman. Virginia snake root tea is given when labor is sluggish, and lady's slipper can help loosen up a rigid cervical opening.

ENERGY-GIVING HERBS

If your contractions seem to be going on forever and wearing you out, herbal remedies can help. The shock tea mentioned above is a great source of energy. Sip grape juice for strength. Ginger tea is a specific for the female organs, and it is a stimulant. It can increase your energy, but some herbalists warn that it could perhaps increase the possibility of hemorrhage if taken too close to the time of actual birth, because it brings blood to the uterine area. Some people take ginseng to give strength during labor. The extract is the most usable form. Some women have reported that they just fall asleep during labor, their contractions slowing or stopping, and when their bodies have received enough energy and rest, labor resumes forcefully and the baby is born. You might mix up "laborade," a rough parallel to the intravenous solutions that are administered in hospitals and similar to the electrolyte drinks that are sold commercially. It is made by mixing 1/3 cup lemon juice, 1/3 cup honey, 1/4 teaspoon sea salt, and 1 crushed dolomite tablet into enough water to make one quart. This is a good mixture for restoring energy and also for taking after vomiting, such as during morning sickness. It is good for giving children instead of the commercially-available Pedialyte solution, which is not of a particularly high vibration. It is also an excellent substitute for Gatorade, both for athletes and for children with diarrhea

PAIN

If you experience discomfort which crosses the threshold into pain, you may feel resentment toward all those ladies who insist that childbirth is not really painful. Some of our pain is caused by fear and tension, and coaching by our birth attendant can help ("Relax your neck, relax your legs," etc.). Many women claim that the relaxation of their mouth directly affects the dilation of the cervix! Having learned Lamaze breathing for my first birth, and having hyperventilate, I have come to prefer the Bradley method of labor, where you try to go limp, breathe softly in the abdomen, speeding up the breathing when it becomes necessary, but not locking into any particular form of breathing. You really need an intuitive and skilled labor coach to guide you into the appropriate breathing. Pressing the appropriate zones on the feet and hands has removed most of the pain from my labors; but if you have someone press your heel zone, he must have much strength and endurance to meet the demands of your contractions. Pressing the right ankle during birth is easier and, for me, very effective, although midwives have told me that some women cannot bear the pressure on their ankles. By far the most effective is using the combs on the heels of the hands. This is extremely relaxing and pain-relieving. One practitioner warns, however, that if you choose this method, you should not practice the technique too vigorously in the weeks just before you are due, because it is so effective that it has been known to start labor. Some laboring mothers appreciate pressure on the sacrum or femoral bones. I have always found these very irritating, but they might be worth a try.

Some herbs effectively cut the pain of birth. You can use tincture of lobelia if your attendant is skilled with it; too much can cause vomiting and actually retard labor. Some midwives say that a lobelia enema cuts the pain by half. In early labor, when the contractions ache like menstrual cramps, motherwort tincture can take off some of the pressure. Use 3-5 drops in water as needed. Skullcap and/or St. John's wort work well for cutting the pain.

At The Farm, the midwives seem to give ladies who are experiencing a good deal of pain a little lecture, telling them to pull themselves together and handle the contractions better. Knowing the suggestibility of laboring ladies, I am sure that this works.

I also like to nurture a feeling of gratitude and love for my husband, my midwife, my baby-to-be, and especially for Christ during birth. I remember that He suffered much worse than what I am going through, and I look to Him for the strength I need. Of course, different religious beliefs could affect the way you approach this love-thankfulness approach, but it's a good one and a real help during the hard times of labor.

On the day I was to go into labor with my fifth child, Avi, my friend, a very busy woman, had decided to come over to check out the location of herbs, materials, etc. After we had discussed the whole routine, my water broke all of a sudden and I went into labor! We called the university to bring Avraham home, and couldn't locate Diane, the midwife, so we called her back-up attendant, Gloria, who was out on her farm at the moment! I went to bed, with my friend doing my hand zone and encouraging me. When Avraham arrived, he took over my hand and my friend worked on my ankle. Baby Avi, who was very large in the womb, caused a strong and intense labor, but the feeling in the room during the whole experience was holy and angelic, and I felt full of gratitude for everyone and everything. He was the only baby I could feel descending the birth canal, and after his head was born, his shoulders and then his torso got stuck, necessitating much hard pushing. He weighed 9-1/2 pounds, where the rest of my children had weighed more or less 7 pounds!

Your attendant will help you to know when you can push; some people think that if the urge to push is very powerful, then it must be time to push. Others say that an internal check is mandatory at this point, because if the os is not fully dilated, pushing can cause it to be puffy and inflamed and slow down the actual birth process. We usually opt for the internal check.

When you're pushing, don't be afraid to grunt or moan or call out. The feeling of pushing out a baby can be the most intense experience you have had, and vocal sounds are fine. I have screamed during this pushing time, not because of pain so much as the intensity. Talk this over with your husband and attendant beforehand so they don't try to hush you inappropriately.

They will be watching when the baby descends the birth canal, which you may or may not be able to feel clearly. When the vaginal opening bulges and the top of the head appears, they will probably tell you to stop pushing. Supporting the perineum, they will ask you to pant or perhaps push gently as the head emerges. When it does, they will immediately check for the cord around the neck; if it is there, they will likely be able to pull it either around a shoulder or off the top of the head. They'll let you know when it is time to expel the rest of the baby, which usually happens in a swift swoosh.

Some claim that whenever possible, the husband should be the one to catch the baby, as it completes the cycle of love. It is a moving and sacred experience for the husband to accept his wife's gift of love and I recommend this practice if you can arrange it.

After the baby has emerged, the midwife or doctor will usually examine it carefully to make sure that it is generally fine. They will ensure that it breathes right away and changes from a usual bluish color to a nice pink. When they are sure it is all right, they will likely place it on your tummy for you to love and hold until the cord stops pulsating. Be sure to cover the baby with a receiving blanket, because it is going from 98.6 degrees inside you to about 70 degrees room temperature, and it is wet besides. Your body warmth will help it maintain.

The cord should stop pulsing completely before it is clamped and cut. Usually a clamp, or tie, which must be tied very carefully and tightly, is placed an inch away from the navel and another placed similarly two inches from the first; the cord is cut with a sterile scissors between. Sometimes the midwife will clamp the second place with a hemostat. When the baby is washed and dressed, he should be diapered so nothing touches the cord stump. Every time you change him, you should replace the 4x4 gauze pad by cutting a slit in the middle of it, slipping it over the cord stump, and then sprinkling a little golden seal or myrrh powder over the stump. Some people use alcohol for this purpose, but the herbs are antiseptic and much milder and nicer.

You may want to bathe the baby in a good, warm bath as with the Leboyer method; this is especially good if the baby seems tense. The bathing can help stabilize baby's breathing. The midwife or doctor will suction out mucus if needed. Watch the newborn carefully for about twelve hours to make sure s/he is breathing well.

EXPELLING THE PLACENTA

Nursing the baby will stimulate contractions, facilitating the expulsion of the placenta. Some attendants get nervous and consider transporting the mother to the hospital if the placenta doesn't deliver right away. We have been comfortable waiting forty-five minutes, even an hour, before the characteristic gush comes and the contraction with it that delivers the plancenta. Your birth attendant should be able to ascertain your condition. No one should tug on the cord to help the placenta deliver, because this could tear it and cause hemorrhage. When the placenta delivers, your attendant should check it thoroughly, because if any of it is retained, you can develop a high fever and endanger your life. You might like to look closely at it, to learn a little what a healthy placenta should be.

I like to shower after birth, but some women bleed overmuch if they get up, and some feel too weak to walk around right after birth. Don't bathe. Someone might give you a bed bath, which will feel wonderful if you sweated during the birth. Your attendants or husband will make your bed fresh for you.

If the placenta does not expel for along time, take a cup or two of red raspberry tea, sweetened with honey. Nurse the baby or otherwise stimulate the nipples, as this powerfully contracts the uterus. Some midwives use ground ivy, catnip, basil, or Dong Quai to help expel the placenta. If the placenta still doesn't expel, and you feel a concern, you can always go to the hospital; if the situation really warrants it, don't feel bad about going.

HEMORRHAGE

If you experience hemorrhage, which is defined as more than two cups of blood, either seeping slowly or gushing out, the first thing you should do is work the uterus externally, kneading the belly until the uterus maintains its shape. This may take some time, but continue until it works. Mistletoe leaf tea of blue cohosh tincture or oxytonic may help clamp down the uterus. Motherwort tea is claimed to help. Most midwives I have met swear by shepherd's purse, best used as a tincture. This humble garden weed is a powerful styptic, although it should not be used routinely as it can cause large, painful blood clots. In hemorrhage it is said to work every time. I consider the shock tea an excellent anti-hemorrhage remedy, although controversial. Local midwives trust cayenne and use it extensively. Cayenne does not contract the uterus; it merely controls bleeding. You might combine it with blue cohosh for both activities.

SHOCK

Some women go into shock after the birth of a baby. In addition to the shock tea, you might take some of the Bach Rescue Remedy; I have used it and found it very effective. Lobelia is also said to be good for shock.

PERINEAL HYGIENE

Every time you use the bathroom, you should flush the perineal area with a combination of a pint of warm water and a tablespoon of tincture of green soap, which is inexpensive to buy at pharmacies. This is a disinfectant and will prevent bacteria from entering your body. Always wipe from front to back. If you have torn or feel puffy or sore around the birth area, comfrey leaf tea, taken internally and used as a wash over the area should speed healing. Fresh aloe vera will heal and relieve pain. Be sure to use a fresh sanitary napkin each time you use the bathroom. Use the underpads as long as you are bleeding strongly; usually the baby's nursing will bring gushes of blood out and completely soak sanitary napkins, clothing and the underpads.

AFTERPAINS

Even more than labor and birth, I have developed a dreadful panic about afterpains. I have them so intensely that, every time the baby nurses, I nearly go into shock--clamminess, shaking, and real pain.

Midwives have suggested St. John's wort, mistletoe, rice bran syrup and calcium tablets, which did not even touch the pain. I tried Lamaze-type breathing without success. The usual pain-relieving herbs, such as catnip or valerian, had no effect. Finally, I purchased some cayenne tincture (hot!) and tincture of lobelia. I put a big squirt of each, which is a lot of both under normal circumstances, into a cup of diluted grape juice, which I drank every time I felt the pains or started to nurse. This, along with applications of Professor Cayenne's Deep Heating Balm, which was really hot and which stained my underclothes, kept the afterpains in control--but just barely! They last for three full days. I was grateful to have the cayenne and lobelia--but more grateful when the pains finally stopped.

I have discovered that the body gives definite signals about what you should be doing after the birth, despite the glorious euphoria that makes you think you are full of energy. For the three days or so that you experience afterpain and bleed heavily, you should stay in bed as if you were ill; this is the body's signal that you need peace and quiet to heal. For the several weeks that follow where you are passing lochia, the blood-like discharge that cleanses the body after birth, you should regard yourself as "on hold." Someone else should do the marketing, the library trips with the children, the heavy chores. You need to adapt to the many, heavy changes that your body is undergoing, changing from a pregnant woman to a lactating mother. You and the baby both need these times of peace and recuperation. I don't know the validity of the claims that primitive women birth in the fields and then get up and continue to work. If we try to emulate these models, we will end up sick in bed and unable to function for much longer than if we take it easy.

After the birth, you should continue taking the green drink, especially the comfrey. If it is winter, comfrey tea will work. This herb contains a cell proliferant that will help rebuild your body. You might also take yellow dock and dandelion tea--together they create a good mineral balance--to build up your blood. The tinctures of both of these are also good for the purpose. Make sure that your diet contains lots of live raw foodstuffs.

ENGORGEMENT

If you nurse your baby right away after the birth, you should have no problems at all with nipple soreness, engorgement, or breast infection. With my first baby, where I was not allowed to nurse for many hours and then encouraged to limit feeding time, I suffered terrible engorgement and sore nipples. With my other babies, as I nursed them consistently right after birth, the nipples responded comfortably and I did not engorge, although for a day or two my breasts seemed quite full. After a while, the milk supply seems to diminish, although it doesn't actually go down.

BREAST INFECTION

If you do happen to get a breast infection, herbal remedies are extremely quick to act. Dr. Christopher's daughter, Ruth, told the story of nursing her baby during a hot night, so she left the window open. A cold breeze came in during the night, and since she had not covered up very well, the cold air blowing on her gave her a cold in the breast. It was very hard and sore, to the point that she could hardly nurse the baby. She tried until she felt like screaming. She called her dad, then about eighty miles away, who came with the mullein/lobelia fomentation. She made it up and covered her breast with it, as hot as she could stand it, and put some plastic over it and then a towel. By morning she was nursing the baby again, with no pain and no more hardness.

Some women use a hot compress of parsley herb, but this can cut down the supply of milk. A hot compress of comfrey leaves, or of marshmallow roots are excellent; the latter is especially good to draw out poisons and infection. Echinacea and garlic can help up an infection; take these internally. My midwife has suggested that a calcium imbalance in the system can cause breast infection; instead of taking calcium tablets, take Dr. Christopher's calcium formula, which consists of four parts comfrey root, six parts horsetail grass, three parts oat straw and one part of lobelia. This can be taken in tea, tablets, or capsules. Take lots of liquids, take hot baths, and be sure to get plenty of rest. Many breast infections result from an exhausted mother. Vitamin C-rich foods, such as rose hip tea or, my favorite, hot lemon toddy, which you make by squeezing the juice of one lemon into hot water and adding honey to taste, can help heal you up.

If your nipples get sore, you can rub on pure lanolin, available at pharmacies. You can sun your breasts briefly, but be careful, because the tissue is tender and sensitive. Honey, comfrey ointment, wheat germ oil, and aloe vera leaf can all be applied, although you should be careful to wash off the honey, as no infant should take raw honey for it may harbor spores which cause infant botulism (see page 93). Remove the aloe vera, because it is very bitter.

Take plenty of time to rest up, to read to the other children if you have them, or to read yourself! Bask in the energy of having a brand new soul in the home. We have babies relatively few times in our lives, and the feelings that accompany a newborn in the home are like nothing else. Heal and enjoy the blessing!

THE NEW BABY

What are the needs of a newborn? After being examined for any defects, cleaned, dressed warmly, he needs two things: to be in close and constant touch with his mother, and to be fed her milk. You might have read the studies on bonding, which show that infants who maintain constant closeness with their parents develop much stronger relationships with them. Writers compare humans with animals; if a mother deer is drugged at birth and doesn't see her fawn within a certain time period, she rejects the baby. Contrary to popular belief, babies can see; I know they can, for my babies look at me and my husband when they are born. Why do people insist that they cannot see? It is because of the use of powerful drugs in the babies' eyes.

SILVER NITRATE

Most states require by law that a baby born in institutions receive silver nitrate drops in order to prevent gonorrheal blindness. For those of us who are faithful in their marriages and who know there is absolutely no danger of venereal disease, this treatment is an insult. If there is a possibility of infection, both the mother, the father, and the doctor can be checked for gonorrhea close to the due date; if they are free from infection, they might be able to waive the silver nitrate. The Lancet, the British Medical Journal, spoke out against the routine use of silver nitrate drops for newborns. The article claimed that the drops are not always effective and could lead to chemical conjunctivitis (and/or blindness). In addition, silver nitrate has no effect against chlamydial infection, the most common venereal disease today. Some doctors offer the use of antibiotics such as penicillin, but this can promote penicillin-resistant gonorrhea germs and develop a sensitation to penicillin. Tetracycline, another antibiotic, is not proven to prevent gonorrheal blindness, nor does erythromycin, a similar preparation. If you do have a hospital birth, do what you can to prevent this eye treatment. If a baby is found to have a gonorrheal eye infection he usually must undergo antibiotic treatment for it anyway, so the initial treatment is superfluous. Any eye infection that develops within a week should be treated by a physician, as gonorrheal infections develop within that time and can be successfully treated. If you are fortunate to have your healthy baby at home and you know there is no chance of infection, you should not concern yourself.

If your baby has an eye infection which is not gonorrheal you can suspect a plugged tear duct. Many mothers gently massage the area and/or wash it with eyebright and golden seal tea, which sometimes helps open the duct. If you choose to massage the area, use very clean fingers. One eye doctor demonstrated: it looks like you're poking your baby in the eye! Press into the inner corner of the eye, then down to the nose. Be gentle and careful but press well. If it doesn't open after a couple of months, you may wish to go to a good eye doctor for surgical opening of the duct. We had to resort to this with one of our sons; the operation was quick and the baby didn't even cry, but it is the last resort.

CONJUNCTIVITIS

Some babies--and children--get pinkeye or conjunctivitis. To treat this eye infection a warm pack of chickweed or teas of red raspberry leaf or eyebright and golden seal, meticulously strained through sterile muslin, can be used to wash the eye. Some midwives suggest flooding the eyes with mother's milk, which contains antibodies. I have tried this with my seven-year-old, who had caught a neighborhood infection of pinkeye. I flooded his eyes with my milk several times a day, and his infection cleared up fast. He thought it was pretty funny, too.

After you know that you have a normal, healthy baby, you must meet his first needs--comfort and food. Both are supplied with breastfeeding. It's a pity that we live in times that are so complex; in former time, mothers had to choose to give their babies this most superior nutrition, because formulas were not available. If mothers did not nurse, they gave their babies to another woman to "wet-nurse."

FORMULA

You probably know there is a strong movement among medical circles to convince mothers that formulas can adequately replace breast milk if the mother chooses not to nurse. Doctors sometimes say that breast milk is deficient in iron, fluoride, or vitamins. Cow's milk is meant to build the bones and muscles of a calf, and its casein content is several times higher than that of human milk. Formulas and canned milks have almost all proven to contain lead, either from processing or from the solder used in sealing the cans. Some formulas lack vitamin B-6, the absence of which causes convulsions. All formulas lack the micro-nutrient, enzymes and life force that mother's milk contains.

EARLY NURSING

Researchers at Brigham Young University have shown that a baby's blood glucose begins to drop at birth, but that a baby who is nursed immediately after birth regains a normal level of blood sugar right away. The longer nursing is delayed, the more severe the drop becomes, and a baby who is withheld from feeding for eight hours or more suffers severe hypoglycemia which is very difficult to recover from. These researchers recommend the obvious and natural prevention: let mothers who wish to nurse their babies after birth do what they want!

Dr. Camilla Wood of this research team also found that, although breastfed babies take in less volume of milk, they absorb and utilize the milk much better, so they don't need ounce for ounce the way bottle-fed babies do. Mother's milk, she found, is more concentrated at birth, becoming more and more watery as the baby grows, which provides the perfect ratio of nutrients to liquid that the baby needs.

EXCLUSIVE BREASTFEEDING

Dr. Robert Mendelsohn goes against standard feeding advice by recommending that mothers breastfeed their babies exclusively for six months. After that, babies should receive the good, natural foods that the parents eat, ground up appropriately.

NURSING

Statistics show that 95% of all women can nurse their babies if they only will. If you find yourself with problems, questions, or just in need of moral support, contact your local La Leche League. Sometimes you can find it listed in the phone book, sometimes from health food stones, or you can contact La Leche League International, 9616 Minneapolis Avenue, Franklin Park, Illinois 60131, telephone (312) 455-7730. La Leche League will answer questions for you, day or night. Personally, I have found breastfeeding my children so easy that I have never needed much guidance, and if you have enjoyed a good home birth and have the support of your husband and family, you will likely have the same experience.

If you cannot breastfeed your infant, see if you can find a close friend who has an infant to help you feed yours. This is not very common these days, however, and you will more likely be able to locate fresh goat's milk, which is the first choice after breast milk: goat's milk most closely approximates mother's milk of all the domesticated animals.

You may be surprised to learn that even a woman who has lost her milk--or one that never has had a child--can breastfeed a child successfully. La Leche League tells of women who patiently ran a tube of formula by their breasts as an infant suckled, and the insistent stimulation brought milk into the mother. Dr. Christopher reminded us that it requires a certain balance of hormones--estrogens and progesterones--to produce milk. If a woman doesn't seem to be making enough milk, she should balance up her hormones by taking a few capsules of Dr. Christopher's hormone balancing formula. Dr. Christopher taught that to make the proper conditions in the woman's body for producing milk, she should take blessed thistle, also known as holy thistle. Taken in doses of three cups or more a day, women who do not have enough milk--or who have no milk--can abundantly supply a baby's needs.

A very unusual lady, blonde, dignified and queenly-looking was planning to adopt a baby and wanted to nurse it. Dr. Christopher told her to go on the mucusless diet, drink a gallon of distilled water each day, which is very necessary because so many people are dehydrated, and to drink three or more cups of blessed thistle tea a day. She planned to receive the baby in a couple of weeks.

One blizzardy day, this lady came into the office, wearing a purple robe with a white fur collar on it. She shook the snow off and was admitted to Dr. Christopher's office. She threw back the robe, and there she had in her arms, at her breast nursing, a beautiful little Navajo baby. She was so blonde that the contrast was amazing. She said she took the baby and put it to her breast, and it started nursing right off. She had taken the blessed thistle tea a few days before the baby was received. Although she had adopted three other Indian children, she felt very close to this one and felt it was a part of her because it was receiving her own milk.

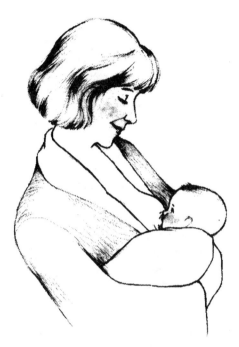

Another time, a young lady in her upper teens came to Dr. Christopher's office asking for help. Her older sister was in a fatal automobile accident and left a newborn baby, thrown out of the car but not hurt because it had fallen in a pile of leaves. The baby would not drink any formulas or anything else. The girl wanted to nurse the baby, although she had never been married nor had anything much to do with men. She drank plenty of the blessed thistle tea, and started nursing the baby within twenty-four hours. She was able to nurse that baby until weaning time.

Our goat got mastitis and recovered, but she lost all of her milk. Normally that would be the signal for breeding her again, but we got a bottle of blessed thistle tablets and fed them to her; they tasted good to her, and she ate them out of our hand. In a day, she regained her high level of milk production (about a gallon a day), which she has maintained for a year and a half, quite unusual for a milking goat.

How often should you nurse your baby? As often as s/he needs it;

you'll be able to tell when the baby is hungry. Use nursing for comfort as well as for nourishment; the more the baby nurses, the more milk you'll make (and the longer you will remain infertile, if you're nursing exclusively). Don't begrudge the time you are nursing; if you have other children you can read to them during nursing time, and you also can use the time to read things you have been waiting to get to. Relax, enjoy yourself. We sometimes forget that babies are tiny for a very short time, really. In several months that tiny one will be wiggling out of your arms, wanting to get down and explore the world. Enjoy his/her softness and cuddliness while you can.

How long should you nurse your baby? Ideally, a baby should wean him/herself, usually after at least a year and preferably two years. Some children want to nurse longer. Sometimes a child will stop nursing and then want to resume when a new baby arrives, or when there is sickness or accident.

Especially when a mother nurses a baby for a long time, she may reach points where she thinks she doesn't have enough milk or that her milk isn't "rich" enough to satisfy the baby. Most infants go through growth spurts when they need a sudden increase in nutrition to satisfy their needs. The first and easiest remedy for this is to nurse more often and longer. You can take the blessed thistle to increase the volume of your milk; marshmallow and red raspberry leaf teas are said to enrich the content of the milk. When I am nursing a baby full-time, I take a nap every day. I put the older children in charge of the younger ones, put the baby to the breast, and go to sleep for at least an hour. An exhausted mother cannot produce adequate milk for her baby. Dr. Christopher stressed the importance of drinking at least a gallon of steam-distilled water every day; he said that most individuals are dehydrated. You will find a big difference in your overall feeling--and your milk production--if you drink enough. Some women recommend taking a tablespoonful of brewer's yeast in juice (apple juice goes well with the flavor) to increase milk. If you ask around, you can find a good-tasting yeast. I find that this remedy really does increase milk yield, and it brings up the blood sugar and gives stamina to a harassed mother. Start with a smaller dose and increase gradually to avoid the possibility of gas for you and/or colic for the baby.

Don't give in to the warnings that your breast milk might be deficient in essential nutrients for your baby. If you are following the mucusless diet, including a variety of fruits and vegetables, you will be getting all the nutrition both of you need. God engineered breast milk to satisfy the needs of your infant. He also supplied immunity to disease through the antibodies from the immune system of the mother. It establishes appropriate intestinal flora, which can be a benefit throughout the child's life. Breastfed babies experience a low incidence of Sudden Infant Death Syndrome, although it sometimes does happen. Breastfeeding helps the infant excrete dangerous substances: when babies are exposed to radioactivity, the breastfed babies excrete twice as much of the substance as bottle-fed babies similarly exposed. Breast milk does not harbor these substances, but cow's milk does (*The People's Doctor*, Vol. 9, No. 12, p. 7)

WEANING

In other cultures, prolonged nursing is acceptable and natural. We should be willing to set aside our cultural expectation and give the little ones what they need. Gradual self-weaning is best. Dr. Christopher recalled the weaning feasts mentioned in the Old Testament; weaning is a special and sacred time. Hannah nursed little Samuel until he was ready to leave home and go to live in the temple!

Probably the best weaning food, in my opinion, is slippery elm gruel. It is smooth, healing, easy to digest, and cuts mucus from the system. When you prepare it, mix a teaspoon of the powder with cold water, add hot waster until it is a gruel, and sweeten with maple syrup, not honey. Honey should not be used by babies until they are a year old. Slippery elm gruel is also a good remedy if the baby has colic or diarrhea.

I have found that my babies exhibit a desire to eat from around six to eight months. We just grind up fruits and vegetables, and later grains and proteins, in our baby food grinder. I also give water and juices by cup and sometimes in a bottle. Dr. Christopher said that the coming in of the first teeth signals the ability to digest food; the eye teeth and stomach teeth indicate that the baby now has gastric juices to handle foods, but we find that our babies demand feeding some time before that!

SERIOUS ILLNESS

Don't be falsely comforted, however, that totally breastfed babies cannot get seriously ill; they do. However, they will enjoy greater protection than bottle-fed babies. Our last child, Sarah, got the flu when she was five weeks old; the flu went into pneumonia, which we had never experienced in our family before. She turned grayish-blue, went limp, and could not nurse. We had to rush her to the hospital, where she was given oxygen and intravenous fluids, including antibiotics. This was the first time we had ever used the hospital for any ailment in our family; it was terribly stressful. But it did show us the true use of hospitals: excellent treatment in times of emergency. As soon as we could, and it took a little arm twisting of the doctor, we took Sarah home. For two months we had neck adjustments and adjustments by a chiropractor who understood the maladjustment of the pyloric and ileocecal valves and taught us to adjust them. We had daily hot baths together, every other day giving a thorough accupressure massage on the feet. We gave finely-minced garlic three times a day in acidophilus. We administered tinctures (which we determined she needed through the chiropractor, who used applied kinesiology). We stayed home during the long, cold winter months. This grueling procedure yielded results: after two months, Sarah lost the purple rings under her eyes, she fattened up, and became strong and vital again.

YEAST INFECTION IN BABIES

I had undergone a stressful pregnancy, not from family problems but because of a neighborhood situation. I attribute Sarah's weakness and susceptibility to my stresses when she was in the womb. At birth, she had a lot of thrush in her mouth, which carried through her system to become a very stubborn yeast diaper rash. Looking back, I would count the presence of such yeast infections as a dangerous signal, because I believe that a body so invaded by yeast is very vulnerable to disease. If your baby has thrush, which you can determine from white spots on the sides of the mouth, a white tongue, or soreness during nursing, you can try several remedies. Dip a Q-tip in the antiseptic tincture (an herbal extract found on page 201) and swab the area several times per day, then give raspberry tea in a bottle. Other remedies may include washing the white parts with a Q-tip soaked in yogurt or, from a drugstore, purchase Gentian Violet, which is an inexpensive germicide, not necessarily an herb but an old-fashioned and effective remedy. With a Q-tip dipped into the liquid, don't soak but just coat the infected surfaces. Gentian Violet will stain anything it comes into contact with.

In order to get to the source of the problem, you need to help the baby feel no stress, make sure your own yeast infections are under control (see page 152), and help restore the baby's proper bacteria composition in the intestine. Use acidophilus freely yourself, and give the baby acidophilus, either the liquid or a capsule dissolved in a little sterile water.

JAUNDICE

Many parents worry about infant jaundice, which occurs in an increasingly high percentage of newborns, which some attribute to the use of drugs in the birth process. Although the symptoms are pretty much the same--yellowness in the skin and eyes--there are actually three kinds of jaundice. Physiological jaundice occurs in blonde babies, Native American babies, those born with the aid of drugs, those not allowed to nurse immediately after birth and on-demand, and preemies. This "normal" jaundice occurs in an actively-nursing and otherwise active, normal baby. It disappears within one month. In order to help the baby overcome this jaundice be sure that the baby passes its meconium within the first day, because meconium contains bilirubin which causes this jaundice. Nurse the baby a lot in order to help the meconium pass; if it doesn't come within a day or two, you might need to see a doctor to find if there is something wrong with the baby's eliminatory system. Take the baby out into the sunlight, naked, for a few minutes each day, or let him lie undressed in front of a sunlit window if the weather is cold. Sunlight breaks down bilirubin. Do this every day until the baby's color is normal. Catnip, comfrey and dandelion tea are said to be good for relieving the problem; drink them yourself, and offer a few drops, from an eyedropper, to the baby; however, do not give any honey to a small baby! Honey can be diluted, processed or come from an environment that is toxic or from weakened, sugar fed bees and often contains botulism spores, harmless to older people, but dangerous to infants, who can contract infant botulism. Also babies are sometimes unable to handle the concentrated sweetness of honey, which can bring on various symptoms, sometimes even death. Our little Sarah, during the week following her hospitalization, passed out when we gave her a bottle of tea, sweetneed with honey; it took her a long time to recover, and this terrible lesson convinced me that no baby should receive honey. Use pure maple syrup if you feel something must be sweetened; I simply give her herbs unsweetened, and she did just fine. As a side note, I believe the best form for giving herbs to a small baby is in a glycerite, the next best being the tincture or extract form. We gave Sarah dandelion extract, along with yellow dock, catnip, marshmallow, and others, and I believe they were extremely helpful in healing her. Three drops of tincture or extract can equal a full cup of tea for a little one; it is much easier to administer.

Doctors admit that another form of jaundice, breast milk jaundice, is extremely rare. Doctors say that this jaundice is also not life-threatening. You can stop breastfeeding for a day, or at the most two, if you wish, but I would just keep taking dandelion for the liver and supplying milk for the baby. Some mothers take fresh wheat grass juice, giving a few drops to the baby.

Both physiological and breast milk jaundice occur in a healthy, active baby. Neither requires special treatment, and the bilirubin usually goes down after the third day. Many doctors wish to treat these babies with bilirubin lights for these types of jaundice. The dangers of this treatment to babies have been identified as irritability and sluggishness, diarrhea, lactase deficiency, intestinal irritation, dehydration, feeding problems, riboflavin deficiency, disturbance of bilirubin-albumin relationship, poor visual orientation with possible diminished responsiveness to parents, and DNA-modified effects (*The People's Doctor*, Vol. 4, No. 7, p. 2). In addition Dr. James Sidbury of the National Institute of Child Health and Human Development suspects phototherapy might be responsible for increased mortality, particularly in small infants, because of lung problems and hemorrhage.

The only dangerous kind of jaundice is pathological, resulting from an Rh or ABO blood incompatibility, or a damaged or malformed liver, or as a side effect of something wrong with the mother, including drug use. The bilirubin continues to rise after the third day, and the baby becomes dehydrated and lethargic. This unnatural condition can lead to brain damage. As usual, the best way to decide what to do is to watch your baby and follow your maternal intuition. If you feel inclined, do not hesitate to utilize treatment from the medical community for this condition. Milk thistle seed extract, plantain, and dandelion herb plus castor oil fomentations, the three oil massage program, and bone, flesh, and cartilage formula fomentations have been known to produce healing results, but be wise and apply these aides under competent assistance. You can take the herbs listed along with garlic, echinacea, and the liver-gall bladder formula to provide additional aid through your breast milk.

My first baby, hospital-born without drugs but not allowed to nurse until 12 hours after birth, was a little jaundiced. The color disappeared within a week or so. My other children, however, born at home and nursed immediately and as long as they wished, never developed jaundice.

CONSTANT CONTACT

Probably the most important need of a newborn after good breast milk is constant contact with the mother. In a society which forcefully limits the time babies spend with their mothers, insisting on placing them in cribs with toys, music boxes and other contrivances to keep them happy, the concept of the family bed and holding the small infant seem very radical. Yet if you draw back from your cultural preconceptions and evaluate the real situation, you see that God must have intended for babies to be held, for they are completely helpless and also express perfect contentment when they are cuddled close to their mothers. Jean Liedloff, in her book *The Continuum Concept*, describes her time spent living among the Yequena Indians of South America. By far the most important difference between their society and ours was the way mothers treated their babies. From birth, babies remained in constant contact with their mothers or someone else. Usually during the first few months, the mother kept the baby by her, nursing on demand, slinging the baby by her side while he slept during the day, sleeping with him at night, even carrying him with her and nestling him across her knees while she tended the small hut fire during the night. As he grew older, an older child or sometimes the father would carry the baby constantly, although the mother continued to nurse him. When the baby finally started to wriggle down to try crawling around, he was allowed to do so. But when tired, hungry, or hurt, he would make his way back to his mother.

Astonishingly, after that long and constant contact, the baby did not become spoiled and demand constant hugging when he was old enough to get around. On the contrary, Liedloff noticed the remarkable independence of these infants. The parents also nurtured self-reliance, never chiding the little ones if they got too close to danger, such as running water, knives, or deep pits. They trusted their children to take good care of themselves--and the children did.

I have always picked up my babies when they cried, and we often slept together, but I never applied the concept of the family bed--where the babies sleep right with the parents during the first year or two--until my sixth baby. I found that this baby was much more independent, when she began to crawl, and much more trusting of other members of the family who held her and tended her. Furthermore, and to my great surprise, I truly enjoyed having her in bed with us, even though she wiggled and kicked like any little baby. I carried her around constantly before she wanted to get around herself, and although I cannot quite agree with Liedloff--"Baby care is nothing to do"--because cutting carrots, scrubbing a floor, and carrying a hot pot are all very much complicated by having a baby in your arms, I still find the investment in my little one worth it, and I recommend the practice to all new mothers. You can buy or make baby slings to help the process. When you consider that our cuddly new baby will only live in your arms six to eight months, carrying her/him will not seem so interminable. You can share the cuddling with siblings or your spouse. Liedloff postulates that many of the aberrations appearing in our society such as drug abuse, alcoholism, inappropriate sexual behavior, thievery, and worse, could be linked to the absence we experience of feeling "right" in our mother's arms. Perhaps during meditation and self-searching we can determine the accuracy of these ideas in ourselves and thus be more committed to help our babies feel safe and right.

Observing my own and other babies, I think that something nourishing passes between a mother and her infant. Babies who live in institutions, fed but not cuddled, fail to thrive and sometimes die, lacking this very real but invisible something. Mothers benefit from the flow of love as well as babies. Sometimes I would wake up in the night to see our baby asleep by my side, and feel so grateful that we can have her close to us.

Small babies need to live quietly. I used to take my babies out marketing, to the library, to movies--everywhere, and I still think there is some merit in that. But in the first few months, mother and baby are better off cutting out the nonessentials and staying home together. Let the father or some kindly relative or neighbor do the errands. When you do go out, carry the baby in a front-pack so s/he feels at home.

Babies can be very sensitive to surroundings, and some can become unhappy and upset at too much running around.

CIRCUMCISION

Today many parents are choosing not to circumcise their baby boys, waiting until the boys grow up and make that decision on their own. Medical research indicates that there is no real benefit in circumcision, other than social acceptance by one's peer group. Probably the only real reason left for circumcising boys is religious, but that can be a powerful and positive reason. Much controversy exists about whether this operation harms the child's psyche in later life; some insist that it does; others say not. You will want to carefully consider your reasons for circumcising your infant.

COLIC

Probably the worst problem with little babies is colic. Almost every one of my children has had it, more or less. If you carry your little one around constantly, the problem can be somewhat relieved. If you are fortunate enough to live outside, in a tent or other outdoor arrangement, and carry your baby, I predict you'll have little colic, because I believe toxins and tensions melt away out of doors. No one knows for sure what causes the problem. Some say that babies have immature digestive systems. Some think that food allergies in mother or baby might bring it on. A mother's tension and unhappiness could induce it.

There are several approaches to the problem. You can suspect food allergies if the baby is constipated, has dark circles under the eyes, wakes up with a start, often passing gas, has red cheeks, and sweats while nursing. Most people can be allergic to dairy products, wheat, eggs, corn, soy and citrus. You can eliminate these one by one to see if baby improves; it takes about three days to get the food elements from one's system, however. You can eliminate all of them for several weeks and add them back one by one to see if your suspicions are correct.

Certain foods seem to be very gas-forming for breast-fed infants: anything from the cabbage family (cabbage, broccoli, brussel sprouts, kale, radishes, turnips, cauliflower, etc.), onions or garlic, peanuts, and chocolate. Prune juice or laxative herbs can cause cramping in a baby's intestines.

See if your baby needs a chiropractic adjustment; sometimes colic is caused by a malalignment in the spine. This might be indicated if the baby cries even if you love him a lot, hates to lie on his back, seems more coordinated on one side than the other, and sometimes breathes irregularly. Our baby's colic cleared up noticeably when we had her neck put in.

Similarly, sometimes an open or closed ileocecal-caecal valve can cause cramping and colicky pain. A chiropractor can sometimes put this in and teach you how to do it yourself.

Several herbs can help colic. The old standby, which I think is wonderful, is catnip tea. You can make a tea of the leaves and give it by bottle (if the baby will take it; mine never would). You can also give it by clean eyedropper, pausing between squirts to make sure that baby takes it. The catnip and fennel tincture works wonders in a colicky baby, and it is so mild that you can feel confident in giving it as needed. If you are uncomfortable with the alcohol content, drop the dose into a spoonful of boiled water and let the alcohol evaporate; then give the dose by spoon. You can also make or buy catnip and fennel glycerite, which is perfectly safe to give as needed. It is sold as Kid-E-Col. In ten minutes or so the cramping should cease and the baby cheer up. In England, dill water used to be the standard treatment for colic; you could buy it commonly in pharmacies. Dill seed tea can work to help colic. Although peppermint is quite strong, some babies respond to it. You can rub the baby's spine with tincture of lobelia to help relax him/him, but I would be very careful about choosing to give it internally.

Especially for an older baby, slippery elm gruel is an ideal colic remedy. You mix the powder with a little cold water, then add hot water until it reaches a slippery gruel consistency. Mix in a little acidophilus or rejuvelac if you like. If you want to sweeten it, add a little pure maple syrup, but no honey. Slippery elm absorbs toxins and soothes the intestinal tract. It seems to soak up gases! I have used it for colic with great success, and it also helps eliminate mucus from the system. You'll see it show up in the diapers with its characteristic slipperiness, but there's no problem with that.

Going outside for a walk helps colic in most babies. Some babies like to go for a drive. We found that a bath always helps. Once when we were camping in the heat of July, our baby wouldn't settle down. We all trooped down to the river for a bathe, and dipped her in. She screamed the first day, but soon learned to love these dips, and always stopped crying after them.

If your baby seems very tight in the tummy and won't stop screaming no matter what, boil some water, make catnip tea, strain it well, and with a very clean ear syringe give her/him a small enema, very gently. Use this in extreme circumstances, but it can help stop the pain and bring out the gas.

Most babies stop being colicky after three full months. If yours continues, check more closely into food allergies.

DIAPER RASH

One of the best remedies for diaper rash is to go without diapers! At least you can eliminate plastic pants, if you don't mind a little dampness. Sunshine and air can clear the problem very soon. Dr. Christopher maintained that diaper rash can sometimes be traced to the "non-foods" that the mother eats: dairy, sugar, white flour, refined and chemicalized foods. As mentioned above, yeast infection can sometimes cause a very stubborn and irritated diaper rash. Keep the baby clean after each bowel movement. You can spread garlic oil over the rash. You can use cornstarch, except with yeast infections, as a substitute for talcum powder (known to cause cancer), and slippery elm powder makes a nice baby powder. Be careful to wash diapers only in mild soaps and to eliminate perfumes and other harsh chemicals from the laundry. Commercial products such as petroleum-based oils or salves, with mineral oil, leach into the baby's system, robbing his/her body of vitamins and minerals, especially vitamin E. Dr. Christopher's bone, flesh and cartilage (B F & C) ointment does a great job protecting and healing and Weleda Baby Cream is said to work wonders for diaper rash; both contain only natural ingredients. Mullein oil and plantain oil--or either in ointment form--work well to soothe baby's sore bottom.

If the baby develops a yeast infection, you can try to eliminate yeast-containing foods (bread, natural soy sauce, fruit skins, fermented drinks, sweets of any kind) from your diet if you are breastfeeding; this, however, is difficult to maintain. Be sure to give acidophilus or rejuvelac to the baby and to take it yourself. You can use yogurt locally on the rash, but it could sting if there are cracks in the skin. Slippery elm gruel, black walnut, or oak bark could cut off the growth of the yeast.

DRY SKIN, CRADLE CAP

Sometimes baby's skin will dry and crack or crust. Don't use standard baby lotions; they are full of chemicals. The very best approach is to avoid the use of soap, because no baby gets dirty in the first few months of life. Warm water should be sufficient, except when you wash off a bowel movement. Use pure olive oil to lubricate the baby's skin. It cleanses and nourishes.

A lady in Arizona had twin babies, born premature and so small that the doctor was unsure of the best procedure for them. They weighed under two pounds when born, baby girls. They were so small that their little mouths couldn't reach over the nipple to nurse. They refused to take any formulas, so the doctor was at a loss. The lady's mother, the grandmother, said, "Let me take those babies home with me and I will give them olive oil massages. They will come out of this all right." For three or four months, she massaged those babies three or four times a day, from head to toe. They took no oral food at all. They grew extremely healthy with just olive oil massages, and a little water. When they got big enough that they could nurse, the mother having kept her milk in with a breast pump, these babies started nursing from their mother, and grew very rapidly. They became very beautiful. In fact, they won the twins contest in the state fair in Arizona, and their mother, a nurse, was very proud of them.

If you want a special oil for your baby steep flower blossoms, such as roses or lavender, in the olive oil. Let the oil-covered blossoms stand in the sun for a week, then press out while the oil is still warm (you can use the top of a radiator or even the top of a radio for this purpose if it is wintertime). Repeat as desired for the strength you wish. Add comfrey of aloe vera for soothing properties. You can also buy natural baby oils or lotions; try your health food stores, or watch for ads in publications such as *Mothering Magazine*.

If your baby has cradle cap, saturate it with one of these oils at night; in the morning, massage and comb the cradle cap off. I have made oil of rosemary with olive oil, and it worked wonders in removing a stubborn case of cradle cap. You can use the brushes supplied with Betadine Scrubs (from your birth kit) to scrub the scalp. This condition presents no health problems; most mothers remove it just because they don't like the look of it.

COLDS AND FEVERS

Most little babies don't get infections, but it does happen. If a little baby gets a cold or flu, it can go into pneumonia very quickly, so you must watch a sickened baby very carefully. If a tiny infant, one or two months old, develops pallor, irregular breathing, coughing and limpness, you should take it to a doctor right away, because it can mean pneumonia even though there is no fever.

If your infant is exposed to colds or flu, you should treat her/him with garlic and echinacea and follow the procedure for fevers, which follows. Garlic works as an antibiotic and echinacea builds the immune system while also acting as an antibiotic. You can give the echinacea tincture to a very small baby. Put a couple of drops on your breast and baby will get the herbs as s/he nurses. You can give garlic oil to a tiny baby in the same way. If the baby is a few months old, don't hesitate to very finely mince garlic, put it in a little liquid acidophilus or boiled water, and just give it to the baby. It is hot to the taste, so you should "chase" it with a good nursing, to take away the taste. I have full confidence in these two herbs in treating infections.

FEVER

For colds, influenza, or any contagious condition, you can treat a fever at home quite successfully. Just remember that fever can be your friend. It burns the toxins and germs of infection out of the body. The rule is, dry fever is dangerous, but wet fever heals. Therefore, make sure that your child's body remains full of fluid. Avoid dehydration at all costs! Some babies won't take anything much when they are sick, but most babies will accept breast milk. Therefore, be sure that you saturate yourself with plenty of water, teas, juices, broths, whatever you can to make prolific milk. Take blessed thistle, marshmallow root, or brewer's yeast to increase volume. Let baby nurse constantly if s/he wants--and they usually want to. Just give up everything else to keep liquid in the baby until the fever recedes. What a blessing it is to be able to nurse a sick baby who might otherwise take no other liquid!

You can also administer very small enemas, called injections in herbal terminology. Catnip and/or garlic enemas are ideal. My babies hold onto these enemas when they have a fever, absorbing the liquid and medicinal factors. Sometimes I can give three or four of them before any is expelled.

Run a good warm bath, add catnip, ginger, or chamomile tea to it, and get in with the baby. Soak together (nursing if you can) for a long time, adding hot water as necessary, and sponging off with cold water at the end. Babies rehydrate very quickly with this treatment.

Certain herbs help bring moisture to the skin surface, which can help break fevers. Although there are many diaphoretic herbs, my favorites in baby's fevers are catnip, chamomile, peppermint with elder flowers, and echinacea. Your baby will likely reject bottles of these teas, but if your intuition tells you that the baby needs one or more of them, make the tea, strain it well, and give it by eyedropper (extracts can give a more concentrated dosage, but increase the liquids). Your baby will swallow them and you can continue administering them, squirt by squirt, until you feel the dosage is enough. None of these herbs can harm a baby. Repeat small doses every couple of hours. Take cups of the infusions (teas) yourself, as well, to impart the medicinal factors to the child

TEETHING

Some babies develop fever, irritability, rashes, vomiting, and other disorders when teething. I don't understand what happens in the child's system to cause these symptoms. Dr. Christopher suggested that the baby's system could lack organic, assimilable calcium which, when received, should stop the symptoms immediately. You should make sure the child is not dehydrated, following the instructions for fever; breastfeed as often and as much as s/he wants. Some mothers offer cooled teething rings; one mother crushes ice and puts it in a thin washcloth. The baby chews on this to relieve the pain. Catnip and fennel extract massaged into the gums help take off the edge. Some teething preparations are made from oil of cloves, which is a natural remedy for toothache and should help localized pain. Sips of chamomile or catnip tea can give generalized relief of pain. Massage the baby's fingers and toes, which are more or less the accupressure zones for the head. Be loving and patient, and the teeth will come through.

VOMITING

If your baby vomits, you must be very careful to maintain hydration. A baby dehydrates very quickly. You can prepare the Laborade (see index), using maple syrup instead of honey. You can give small enemas of catnip tea mixed with slippery elm. The trick is to make them small enough so that the child retains them. The slippery elm soothes the baby's tract and helps the enema be retained. You can try nursing the baby for less than a minute every twenty minutes. The baby will scream for more, but this procedure might help keep the milk down. A drop or two of tincture of lobelia in baby's mouth can relax the tense muscles that cause vomiting. Sometimes a thin gruel of slippery elm will stay down when nothing else will. Don't overlook the wonderfully hydrating effects of a good, long soaking bath with mother. Put in a gallon or so of strong comfrey or chamomile tea for nourishment as well. You can massage the baby (with olive oil) for nourishment and relaxation. I have found this combination--hot herb bath, cold sponge, and subsequent massage-- a wonderful remedy for teething, fevers, flu, and almost every other baby ailment.

DIARRHEA

If your baby has diarrhea, you can follow the treatment for vomiting. Be sure to clean the baby's bottom really well, applying appropriate remedies if the baby gets diaper rash.

EAR INFECTION

If your baby gets an ear infection, try home remedies before you take him or her to the doctor. Two drops of a garlic extract in olive oil followed by two drops of tincture of lobelia or Dr. Christopher's B tincture, plugged with a bit of cotton, often removes the pain and the congestion. It is important to administer the garlic oil first to avoid the pain an alcohol extract can cause to an inflamed ear. You can rub the lymph glands below the ears with the same preparations, or with oil of mullein and lobelia. Ear infections can be a result of a systemic infection, or they can point to dietary problems, either allergies or too many mucus-forming foods in the other. Examine your own condition carefully when your baby gets sick. If the infection remains acute, take the baby to a doctor you trust. Even if you do not purchase the prescription he offers, he will be able to tell you the exact condition of the ears. Some parents have purchased earscopes with which they can examine their own children's ears.

IMMUNIZATIONS

Most parents face the dilemma of immunizations not long after their babies are born. The medical profession insists that you will become seriously ill if you do not receive immunizations, and they really scare parents into having their babies get their shots. Much research has shown that all immunization are, in one way or another, dangerous and/or ineffective. In particular, the DPT vaccine offers specific problems. The pertussis vaccine is still crude and unpredictable; it can cause brain damage from immunological reaction and toxic effect. Although this has been a subject of hot debate, the American Academy of Pediatrics has taken this stand. In one study involving about 15,000 doses of DPT vaccine, with about 4,000 children included, nine children had convulsions and nine collapsed, about 1 child in 400 suffering reactions. In a study published in Sweden, one out of 3,000 children developed some sort of neurological illness after immunization. "Eight of these episodes represented convulsions, 54 shock, 24 abnormal screaming. Three children had permanent brain damage..." (*The People's Doctor*, Vol. 6, No. 10, p. 2). Some deaths have been reported following pertussis vaccination; four instances of SIDS (Sudden Infant Death Syndrome) were reported in Tennessee in children who had received DPT vaccine within the preceding twenty-four hours. Prolonged fever results, with abscesses at the site of the shot; these abscesses, when cultured, showed streptococcus contamination, as sometimes the vials of the vaccine can be contaminated. Some children go into a coma, some develop strong flu-like symptoms, and some exhibit severe allergic reactions, including respiratory problems.

Even the medical profession asserts that the pertussis portion of the vaccine is only 80% effective. Doctors themselves are very cautious about taking the shots. Pertussis, which is whooping cough, is an extremely difficult disease to diagnose, and it can be treated successfully at home with herbs (see Dr. Christopher's book *Herbal Home Health Care*).

Although diphtheria used to be a serious cause of disease and death, today it rarely occurs. Even when it appears, the immunization does not fully protect sufferers. For example, in 1969 sixteen people contracted the disease in Chicago. One-fourth of these had been fully immunized against the disease, and five others had received one or more doses of the vaccine, two of these showing evidence of full immunity. In another outbreak, with three fatal cases, 14 out of 23 carriers had been fully immunized. (*The People's Doctor*, Vol. 2, No. 4, pp. 1-2).

As for the tetanus vaccine, most doctors insist that we must have booster shots at various intervals in order to avoid lockjaw should we step on a rusty nail or have similar puncture wounds. The tetanus injection has varying degrees of potency and, therefore, is not predictable. Furthermore, too-frequent shots (more than once every ten years) can decrease the body's natural immunological response to the germ. Even with the insistence of the medical profession, almost half of the U.S. population has not received the tetanus vaccine, and yet some of these must have stepped on rusty nails. Where are all the cases of tetanus? Dr. Mendelsohn observed that the cases of tetanus he has treated have resulted not from rusty nails but from malnourishment in derelict characters.

One of our children recently stepped on a very rusty nail. It was a typical puncture wound--deep, no bleeding. We manipulated the wound until it bled, and then applied a poultice of crushed plantain weed, fresh, with slippery elm. The boy slept with this on his foot, and in the morning the pain had receded and there was no swelling or redness. Dr. Christopher has cited cases where an individual has wounded himself, infection has set in, and blood poisoning has begun to streak up the limb. With poultices of fresh plantain even these serious conditions can clear up.

Of more serious and far-reaching concern is polio vaccination. My children have not received any immunizations and my mother, who tries to accept our way of life without too much criticism, kept insisting that they at least receive polio vaccinations. However, Dr. Salk, who developed the killed-polio virus vaccine, testified that most of the few polio cases occurring in our country since the early 1790's were the result of the live-polio vaccine. Of the twenty-one cases of paralytic polio in the U.S. in 1982 and 1983, all were vaccine associated. That means, the only way to get polio in his country appears to be to receive the vaccine or to stand close to someone who had recently been vaccinated. Eight of the cases occurred among vaccine recipients, seven of these two to four months old, having received only one dose of the vaccine! To me, this is simply heartbreaking, injecting a pure and innocent baby with a poison that cripples it for the rest of its life. Six other cases occurred among household contacts with vaccine recipients. Five were parents of babies who had received their first vaccination, and one was a sibling, unvaccinated, four and a half months old. Two of the parents had received partial immunization. Three cases occurred among non-family members, two being children, playmates of vaccinated children, and the third having had contact with a baby-sitter's child who had been vaccinated (*The People's Doctor*, Vol. 9, No. 2, pp. 5-7). Almost all people over 18 years old who have contracted polio have been vaccinated.

Why has polio been so drastically reduced in the United States if the inoculations are ineffective? Doctors point to better hygiene, improved nutrition, and better sanitation. Dr. Christopher repeatedly taught that if we keep our bodies clean, germs cannot infect us, because they are only "garbage collectors" that live in toxic conditions. Even people who have contracted serious diseases, when they clean up their bodies, have been able to leave their wheelchairs. A baby who has been properly nourished in the womb and who continues to receive top-quality breast milk doesn't need poisonous injections to keep him well. Smallpox vaccination can cause real problems, including encephalitis, skin conditions, and even death. Measles vaccination can also cause encephalitis, lack of muscle coordination, retardation, learning disability or hyperactivity, aseptic meningitis, seizure disorders and paralysis of one side of the body. Mumps vaccine does not necessarily immunize the recipient. Pneumonia vaccine recipients had the same amount of disease as non-recipients. Flu shots cause flu-like symptoms in their recipients, as well as not providing protection, and sometimes causing paralysis in older individuals. German measles vaccine lasts for varying amounts of time, thus negating the possible good effects for potentially childbearing women.

Finally, clear-thinking scientists are realizing that immunizations are more than just potentially ineffective or only minimally damaging (although if it's your child who suffers the damage, statistics are no comfort at all). Dr. Robert W. Simpson produced research which suggested that immunization programs may be seeding humans with RNA to form proviruses which will then become latent cells throughout the body. Some of these latent proviruses could be molecules in search of diseases which under proper conditions become activated and cause a variety of diseases, including rheumatoid arthritis, multiple sclerosis, lupus erythematosus, Parkinson's disease, and perhaps cancer (*The People's Doctor*, Vol. 6, No. 12, p. 4). Although Dr. Simpson hedged on these findings when later questioned about them, his original research reflects this correct interpretation. At any rate, it is very likely that injecting viruses into the system should weaken immunologic response and weaken the body's resistance to disease.

Mothering Magazine offers a very complete booklet on immunizations. They also advertise various books and booklets on the subject. *The People's Doctor*, a newsletter devoted to exposing inappropriate medical practice, has covered the subject in many issues; you can write for back issues to *The People's Doctor*, P.O. Box 982, Evanston, Illinois 60204. This research by Dr. Mendelsohn is both complete and easy to read.

There are other reliable sources of information if you want to know about immunization dangers. Check with your naturopath or chiropractor for articles. Two good books are *Immunization The Reality Behind The Myth* by Walene James and *Vaccines: Are they Really Safe and Effective?* by Neil Z. Miller. This latter book is the most up-to-date of any books we have seen, and we especially like the chapter on the long-term effects of vaccination, which suggests that the immune system can be impaired by damage to the thymus gland. Injections of viruses and viral agents can affect your genetic structure, although no one has broad, long-term research on this subject. The AIDS epidemic is linked to polio vaccinations contaminated with SV-40, which is a powerful immunosuppressor and trigger for HIV, the AIDS virus. Other monkey viruses can contaminate polio viruses, but tests for these contaminants have only recently been discovered, and who knows how many more may yet exist? This book also details specific problems associated with each particular vaccine. It is excellent reading for parents who must decide on immunization.

If you decide not to immunize your children, as we have, you can still send your children to school. Most states require that you sign a waiver form, and the school districts can give you a hard time, but you are not legally required to immunize for school attendance in most states. For example, the Christian Scientists the world over are successful in avoiding immunizations and other medical interventions.

From the above, you will see that immunization is a very dubious practice, especially for your pure, new infant. The best protection against disease is good nutrition, regular exercise, pure air and water, and a happy, balanced lifestyle.

When you gaze into a new baby's eyes, you can see evidence of a mature soul or spirit far beyond the smallness of the infant. Some people assume that this is evidence of reincarnation. Dr. Christopher believed that a mature spirit entered into a tiny body, and that the spirit does have intelligence and depth. If you can tune into the personality and spirit of your new baby, you will treat her/him quite differently than if you considered her/him just a helpless little bundle of humanity. Reach into your baby's spirit; quietly observe his attributes. You will see that he understands much of the quiet talk you give him, and you will see the great love he has for you. Treating babies this way is much more interesting and fun than simply taking care of their physical needs and cuddling them, as important as these things are.

Perhaps because of these spiritual aspects of babies, a mother is gifted with special insights into the needs of her little ones. Kitty Frantz said, "Look at your baby. Try to trust your gut-level feeling. I personally think the gut-level feeling is called the Holy Spirit. There's an inner voice you can tap into. I think every mother, no matter where she is in her mothering, has a sense of what she should and shouldn't do.

"Oftentimes I'll say to a mother, 'What do you think is wrong with your child?' She'll answer, 'I think it's his left ear.' And you know what? It's his left ear.

"Shut everything else out and ask your heart, What do I think is wrong? And then try to validate your impressions from this basis" (*Mothering Magazine*, Spring 1986, p. 66).

You will find that mothering children with this state of mind is a glorious and freeing experience. When you need to treat their illnesses, this same intuition will lead you to the right herbs and remedies.

HEALTHY WOMAN

In his book *Male Practice*, Dr. Robert Mendelsohn chronicles the incredible mistreatment of women by medical doctors. He shows the unnecessary drugs, surgeries and other treatments that women are subjected to as they bow to the "god image" of modern medical practitioners. In particular, the number of needless hysterectomies, which he compares to castration, is appalling.

Fortunately, a woman can heal herself--and her loved ones around her--with herbs and natural treatments. As Dr. Christopher proved so often with his Incurables Program, even dreadfully sick people can heal themselves.

Dr. Christopher told story after story about sick women he helped with simple remedies, simple treatments. For example, a man and his wife brought their daughter to Dr. Christopher's office in Salt Lake. This young lady was the sickest, saddest-looking person he had seen in a long while. She had met a young man who came to love her very much, and he wanted to marry her. But she refused, saying it wasn't fair to him, being in her condition, so anemic and sickly. He told her that he loved her enough to marry her and take care of her under any circumstances.

She was in a very serious condition, so they put her on the three-day cleanse and mucusless diet. She took extra cups of red clover combination tea, and drank a minimum of one pint of grape juice a day, chewing each mouthful. When she could, she took even more. She also ate plenty of raisins and grapes in addition to the juice. She used the yellow dock as a tea, and soon she began to show improvement. She exercised adequately, being careful not to overdo it, and changed her diet from mucus-forming food to the mucusless diet, having lots of salads and fruits, emphasizing as much raw food as possible. She used the female corrective and hormone balancing formulas, and she also used the vaginal herbal bolus and yellow-dock combination in the slant board routine. She showed improvement from the very beginning.

The parents had brought her to Dr. Christopher in the spring, and by fall they sent him an invitation to her wedding. She had cleaned up her system and was looking forward to marriage. She was menstruating regularly and had gotten over her case of anemia. She was living a new life, healing herself by following through on Dr.

Christopher's plan.

REPRODUCTIVE SYSTEM

Dr. Christopher always checked his patients with iridology before advising them. A lady came to him, about age 45, asking for a reading to help with her condition. He saw that she had a prolapsed transverse colon which had dropped to a point where it tipped her uterus and pinched her bladder, and she was having very serious trouble there. She had infection in both her ovaries and she was troubled with vaginal drainage. In addition, she had one breast that was badly infected, which might necessitate having part of the breast removed if she asked another doctor for treatment. After the reading, Dr. Christopher asked why she had come to him and what she wanted him to do. She said that she had just spent three days in a clinic, where they had verified everything he had read from her irises, but they wanted her to go to the hospital immediately and have the uterus removed and the bladder stitched up to the spinal cord area, and also have her breast removed. She was frightened of all this cutting, so she wanted to find help in some other way.

She promised that she would stay on the program that Dr. Christopher advised. She took the female corrective and hormone balancing combinations, used the vaginal herbal bolus six nights a week, flushing out each morning with the slant board routine, massaging 15 to 20 minutes a day on the abdominal and pelvic area while the tea was inside. She was also to use the three-oil massage over the abdominal area, and go on the three-day cleanse and mucusless diet. In addition, she was to drink a gallon of steam-distilled water a day, and plenty of red raspberry leaf tea. She kept her bowels clean with the lower bowel formula, her liver clean with the liver-gall bladder formula, her kidneys with the kidney-bladder formula, and the red clover combination to clean her bloodstream (see "Herbal Cleanse" on page 171).

Dr. Christopher did not see her again for six months. When she came to see him this time, she bounced in, not dragging as she had before, a totally different woman, much happier and healthier. She had no operations, and yet her prolapsed transverse colon had returned to its normal place, and her uterus and bladder had gone back into position. She was feeling like a new woman, and she did indeed have a new system by following through with the entire herbal program.

When Dr. Christopher was traveling, using chiropractic offices and naturopath's offices, diagnosing, reading eyes, and helping with herbs, another lady with a similar problem as the above came to see him. In addition to the prolapsed transverse colon infecting the entire reproductive system, it had impinged on the bladder, so that whenever she laughed, sneezed, or coughed, she would void urine, a very embarrassing problem. In addition, one of her breasts was so infected that the doctors were urging her to have it removed.

Dr. Christopher told her he could give her advice as to what to do, but that he was traveling and wouldn't be able to guide her or see her for several months. She agreed to follow his instructions, and asked to see him when he returned.

He put her on the full program. She was to clear the bowel with the lower bowel formula, clear and build her liver with the liver-gall bladder formula, her kidneys with the kidney-bladder formula, take the red clover combination to clean her bloodstream (see "Herbal Cleanse" on page 171), and to rebuild the reproductive organs with the female corrective and the hormone balancing formula. She was to continue the whole program, six days a week.

When he returned to that city six months later, she had called and prearranged an appointment. She came in, looking years younger, all smiles. She said her urine loss was under control now, with no unwanted voiding. She had no pains in the ovaries; in fact, she had dropped some stones during the three-day cleanse. She had also passed some tumors, one almost the size of a grapefruit, and cysts as well. When she went to the family doctor for an examination, he was astounded, because her body was rebuilding itself. The breast they were going to cut off had healed itself, with no more infection. She felt that it was a new world, and that life was worth living again.

Although she healed rapidly and consistently, Dr. Christopher pointed out that herbs don't work all at once. You must apply yourself and patiently wait for the results of your hard work.

A lady who had three children by Caesarean section came to Dr. Christopher because she was "baby hungry." Medical doctors had told her that her scars were so bad that if she dared become pregnant again, the strain on her system would kill both her and her baby. Another section, they insisted, was totally impossible; one doctor crudely said that they couldn't even crochet her back together again if she attempted another pregnancy.

But she wanted another child. Dr. Christopher advised her to begin the usual program with the three-day cleanse once monthly, the mucusless diet, the hormone balancing and female corrective formulas. In addition, he told her to do the three-oil massage, (See "Three-oil massage" in the index). The lady was to sunbathe and exercise as well.

Time passed, and Dr. Christopher had pretty much forgotten about this case. Then one day the lady came to him with a baby in her arms. The scar tissue had begun to soften, and eventually became healthy tissue. She had an easy home birth vaginally, with no complications (VBAC). This lady went on to have other children, grateful to Dr. Christopher for her healing with herbs.

Other herbs used to heal the female system are American angelica, bayberry, beet, bethroot, black cohosh, black haw (anti-abortive), blessed thistle, blue cohosh, boneset, buchu, chamomile, catnip, cedar berries, comfrey, cramp bark, dandelion, elecampane, evening primrose, false unicorn, fennel, fenugreek, feverfew, garlic, German chamomile, ginger, golden seal, gravel root, juniper berry, lemon, lemon thyme, lobelia, myrrh, Oregon grape, parsley root, peach, peppermint, plantain, pleurisy root, prickly ash, red raspberry, rosemary, safflower, sassafras root bark, shepherd's purse, slippery elm, squaw vine, St. John's wort, stinging nettle, thyme, uva ursi, valerian, vervain, white poplar, wild yam (anti-abortive), wintergreen (small), witch hazel, wood betony, wormwood, yarrow.

INCURABLES

A lady called Dr. Christopher in Salt Lake City from Provo, Utah, saying that her daughter had flown in from out of town, extremely ill. She was afraid that she was going to die, so she had come to her mother to be taken care of. The mother asked if he would come and read the young woman's eyes. When he arrived, the young woman ridiculed him, and said she thought it was a bunch of crazy ideas that her mother had, and she wasn't going to let him look into her eyes. So Dr. Christopher bowed out and left.

Nearly a month went by, and the lady from Provo asked him to come again, that the daughter was so sick that she was frightened and would talk with him.

When he came, they told him that they had tried the best doctors they could find, but no one could help the girl (they didn't tell Dr. Christopher what the problem was, however). As he gave her an eye reading she would remark, "Who told you that!" Each thing he told her was the same thing that the doctors had diagnosed. When he finished, she said she was still dubious about the natural program, but that the reading was so accurate, he must have something good. She agreed to follow the natural program. She was too sick to even get up and walk.

So they started off gradually on the Incurables program, using juices to rebuild the body. Before many weeks had passed, she came to Dr. Christopher's classes and became quite a faithful student. She even began to study iridology and became good at it. She watched her own eyes and could see the healing taking place. She had been told, though she had been married for some time, that she could never have a baby because of an immature pelvic area and an underdeveloped uterus, as well as other problems in her reproductive system. By using the mucusless diet and herbs to rebuild her body--the female corrective and the hormone balancing combinations--and doing the exercises they advised, even these problems began to heal.

Eventually Dr. Christopher got a call from her husband on the West Coast; he was angry. It was a call of abuse, accusing the Doctor of keeping his wife up in Utah when she should be down with him. He was an electrical engineer, with a very important job, and felt he needed her with him. Dr. Christopher told him his wife had been too sick to even sit up alone, but with the aid of the program and the mother's assistance, she was improving. He told the husband she would be home with him as soon as possible.

The man told Dr. Christopher he was one of the worst quacks there could possibly be, let out some abusive language, and slammed down the receiver.

The wife did heal eventually, and traveled home on her own, without anyone assisting her. She again had the energy she needed to beautify her home. She showed so much improvement that her husband was astonished, because he had figured she didn't have too much longer to live. Her cure caused a career change for him for although he was an electrical engineer with a high-paying job, he was so delighted with the results that he became a chiropractor.

Best of all, she birthed two beautiful children, naturally and her husband received them in the delivery.

While Dr. Christopher was sitting in his family restaurant that used to be located in the University Mall in Orem Utah, across the hall came the most grotesquely-built wheelchair he had ever seen; it was all out of shape, having been built for someone deformed. And sitting in the chair was one of the most deformed people he had seen. The lady's arms and legs and back were twisted out of shape. She was being pushed by a young lady, who took her right up to Dr. Christopher.

"I am surprised to see you, Dr. Christopher," the lady in the chair said. "I just had to stop and thank you; you have done so much for me."

He began to wonder what the thank-you could be, because she was terribly malformed.

She said that she had been like a vegetable for nearly fifteen years, having to be fed and given liquid to drink. She couldn't even raise a hand or leg. She started on the Incurables program, with some people helping her, and they put the bone, flesh and cartilage fomentation down her crooked back and over other parts of her body--and she said, "Just look at me now."

She was moving her hand, and she raised it off the wheelchair a little bit. She did the same with the other hand. She could turn her head and move her shoulders. She could even move her back a little, although it had not moved for those fifteen years previous. Grateful for her new life, she felt that she would live to get up out of that wheelchair and walk. She was so grateful for the formula. And Dr. Christopher said it would be a wonderful day when this young lady could walk and be on her own after fifteen years.

CANCER

So many people feel that if they have cancer, there is nothing to do but wait and die. Dr. Christopher's program has proved otherwise. I personally have seen cases of diagnosed cancer that have been turned around and the patient become completely well, by faithfully following Dr. Christopher's program (see "Cancer" in index for other case histories).

He had an interesting experience on an airplane. He boarded in Salt Lake City, had buckled up, and was ready to enjoy a little free time on the plane, reading, studying and meditating. A lady sat down beside him. As the plane took off, she began to talk.

"Hello, where are you going?"

"To Toronto, Canada," he replied.

"Why?"

"I lecture, and will be lecturing there."

"What do you lecture on?"

Dr. Christopher could see that he wouldn't be getting much quiet meditation, and began to feel a little irritated, but he answered that he was an herb doctor, lecturing on healing the body.

"Isn't that interesting?' she responded, and began to tell him her story. She said that two years before she had had pains in her breasts, so bad that she went to the doctor. She had severe cancer of the breast, so the physician took her right to the hospital, and when she came out she had only one breast. They assured her that he had cleaned out the cancer very thoroughly, but six months later her other breast started hurting. It got so severe that she again went to the doctor, who said that he must have missed some of the cancer, so he rushed her to the hospital and they removed her second breast. She went home with the assurance that this would be it, no more problems. But within six months, she was having abdominal pains; in her organs and lower cavities, she was in terrible pain. When she was examined, the doctor told her that she would have to have her reproductive organs removed and part of her bowels, because the cancer had spread throughout her body. She said that she wouldn't let them do any more cutting on her. They suggested chemotherapy, but she wouldn't allow that either. She said that if she was going to die, she didn't want to be in pieces. She would die on her own. She went home, not knowing where to turn, knowing nothing about diet, medicine, or anything. She said she knelt down and prayed, and the answer came to her.

Did the Doctor want to know what it was?

By this time, Dr. Christopher was all ears, and yes, of course, he very much wanted to know what it was!

She changed her diet to eat fruits and vegetables, grains and seeds, as much as possible raw. A few months went by and she was feeling better, like a different person entirely. She went back to the doctor, who claimed that she had improved amazingly. There was just a little cancer showing in her pap smear. The doctor said to wait and see what happened. She went back home, and in a few months on this diet of natural foods, she said even the pap smear cleared.

The thought went through Dr. Christopher, "Lord, what kind of a

God are you? It takes me forty years, and this woman kneels down and the answer comes immediately to her! This is exactly what I've been teaching all these years, and learning it gradually."

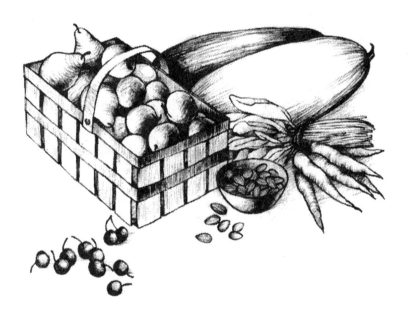

This woman traveled all over the United States, speaking to women's groups, women who fear they might get cancer or women who already have it, telling them to go to live foods and change their diet.

Dr. Christopher felt that their conversation was time well spent!

BONE CANCER

One lady had bone cancer. Her cancerous condition had gone throughout her whole body, but had settled in the bone, and one-and-a-half vertebrae were completely gone. The bone in her body was disintegrated to a point that she could not sit up or walk around anymore; she had to lie in bed. The X-rays showed that the vertebrae above and below the lumbar area were perforated with cancer, so they couldn't even fuse the missing vertebrae to give her support. She had to lie in bed helpless with her little children running around, and a lady coming in the home to help as much as she could.

This lady also had to manage a china shop in Provo, Utah, so she couldn't spend all of her time helping in that home. She called one day, and told Dr. Christopher about the situation. The woman, she said, was just lying in bed waiting for the rest of her spine to deteriorate. Could the Doctor help at all?

He replied that if this woman would follow instructions, there could be some help. The herbs would do nothing but good, and if the woman followed the program in the right frame of mind, she could be healed.

She was started in the Incurables program. The lady needed to clear her bowels with the lower bowel formula, clear and build her liver with the liver-gall bladder formula, her kidneys with the kidney-bladder formula, and take the red clover combination to clean her bloodstream (see "Herbal Cleanse" on page 171). She had to switch from mucus-forming foods to the mucusless diet, and to go on the three-day cleanse every two weeks, in her case. She had to use a gallon of steam-distilled water each day.

Now that the basic body condition was improving, they concentrated on the spine. Before Dr. Christopher came upon the bone, flesh, and cartilage formula, he used comfrey paste for external applications (this paste, comprised of wheat germ oil and honey in equal parts, blended thoroughly and combined with powdered comfrey root or leaf to make a paste, is still super for use on burns, wounds, etc.). They put this paste down the lady's spine, from the medulla at the base of the skull down to the bottom of the tailbone, about four or five inches wide, with flannel over this and plastic over the flannel to keep it from saturating the bed. This was applied each night, six nights a week, week after week. It took a great amount of patience. Many people have gone through this procedure for curvature of the spine, arthritis of the spine, and various ailments, with complete success.

This woman followed through, and in under six months the back was feeling so good that she went back to her osteopathic physician for an X-ray. He said that originally where the bone had been eaten away-- that was one and-a-half vertebrae--the good Lord had healed her.

Cartilage had come in and formed a perfect vertebrae and a half to replace the eaten-away ones--not bone, but cartilage. It gave her enough support that she could get up and take care of her family. At the end of the year, the cartilage had turned to bone, and she had a perfect spine from the top to the very bottom. All that had been perforated formed back solid, and the X-ray showed a spine as good as a teenager's. The physician was astounded! This case proved that even cancer of the bone can be healed with the proper program.

BREAST CANCER

Although many women feel obliged to check their breasts regularly for lumps, and to have X-rays if they suspect anything might be wrong, this approach sometimes can present more problems than help. During 1977, at least 100 women lost breasts unnecessarily because they had been misdiagnosed for breast cancer. Sometimes a cell may appear cancerous under the microscope but behave like a benign tumor. And women who undergo radical mastectomy do not have a better survival rate from cancer than those who have less than radical surgery.

From a natural point of view, cutting out the cancer does not solve the problem, anyway. Cancer appears because there is something basically wrong in the body. Cutting it out may stop it in that particular area for the time being, but it can and does appear somewhere else.

Far better to follow Dr. Christopher's three-day cleanse, mucusless diet, and herbal formulas, such as his red clover combination. Of particular importance is his liver-gall bladder formula, because a healthy liver plays such an active role in combating cancer.

Incidentally, many assert that prolonged breastfeeding helps prevent breast cancer.

Other herbs used to combat cancer are calendula, red clover, wheat grass juice, soaked figs and fig juice, blue violet, parsley, poke root, buckthorn, yellow dock, soaked and ground apricot pits (with their fruit), flaxseed, garlic, chaparral, burdock root, licorice root, echinacea, pau d'arco.

Many have had excellent results taking regular doses of carrot juice, perhaps mixed with celery and red beet juice. Exercise is paramount to recovery and swimming is indicated as the best exercise for diminishing cancer in the breast.

MULTIPLE SCLEROSIS

A young woman in London was put in a wheelchair with multiple sclerosis. She was completely disabled and expected to spend the rest of her life this way.

However, she began to change her diet' she ate fruits and vegetables, grains, nuts, and seeds, some cooked and some raw. She gave her body the nutrition and most essential rest it needed to repair. After a period of months, she was able to get up out of her wheelchair. She became completely healthy and normal, and started to teach other women this process of healing for whatever problems they had. In particular, there were five cases of diagnosed cancer of the cervix. Using the mucusless diet and the vaginal herbal bolus, these five cases were turned around; four were pronounced cleared by the medical profession and the other in remission.

INFLUENZA

A lady called Dr. Christopher when he was in Great Falls, Montana. A patient of his, she was really worried because a couple of their children had come home from school with the stomach flu. This particular flu was spreading very rapidly; when people get it, the whole family gets it. She had eight children--and only one bathroom!

He answered, "The last time I was over at your house, I noticed you had a large patch of red raspberries."

"Yes, but what has that got to do with the stomach flu?'

"Go out and gather several bushels of leaves of the red raspberry bushes; don't rob any of them, but just take a little off each bush. Make it up into a tea. Take a big handful and pour a pint of boiling water over that portion and let it steep for twenty minutes. Make up gallons of it. For the children that have already come home with the flu, give them some as well, and you and your husband, too. If they're hungry, give them this tea. Give them lots and lots of it."

The lady was willing to try anything. And the next time he saw her, she was very happy. She said the two children that had come home sick, just like the rest of the children, might have been out of school for days, maybe weeks. Yet they went to school the next day, along with the rest of the children. She and her husband didn't catch flu, either. Red raspberry tea cleared the sick ones and kept the others from getting sick.

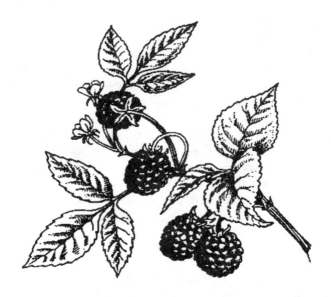

This lady was so enthused about herbs that she decided to study more about herbs. She continued to study, but continued to have her family as well, so that by the time the last one was weaned, she had sixteen children. She then went back to school, to Brigham Young University in Utah, where she got her degree as a registered nurse. She served as a nurse, helping other people.

Once, one of Dr. Christopher's students had broken his leg and was lying in the hospital, in a great deal of pain. The curtain opened, and a little lady put her head through; she had a white nurse's cap on. She said, "You broke your leg? If you want to get healed fast, use lots of comfrey tea."

The student said, "You must know Dr. Christopher."

"Shush," smiled the lady, "Yes I do, but don't tell anybody. I might get fired."

Dr. Christopher's son David used the raspberry leaf tea and cleared an impending case of flu in just one day. He was so delighted that he took his wife out to dinner--and they ate the wrong things. His flu came back strong as ever the next morning. He tried the raspberry tea again, but it didn't work. So he had to use the anti-plague formula which, he said, tastes so nasty that any self-respecting germ will leave just because of the unpleasantness.

Other herbs used for flu include bayberry, boneset, motherwort, pennyroyal, peppermint and elder flowers, pleurisy root, and garlic.

GALLSTONES

Dr., Christopher used to give thirteen lectures a week, in six or seven different towns throughout Utah. During a lecture in Ogden, one of his students, a lady, came to him, saying she was in terrible trouble. She had gallstones so bad and painful that her doctor would give her pain shots. The doctor now refused to give any more shots, but if she had another attack, the stones would be removed.

Another attack was starting, and the doctor told her that an operation to remove the stones would cost $1200. "I haven't got the money," she told the doctor. He said to put it on the medical credit card, which she didn't have either. He said that he couldn't help her until she had the money for the operation.

Then she remembered about the three-day cleanse that goes with the mucusless diet. You use apple juice for three days, as well as olive oil, a couple of spoonfuls three times a day. She decided to try it.

After about a week, Dr. Christopher returned to Ogden. This lady came bouncing through the door, with no pain at all. "Hello, doctor," she said, "I am so glad to see you. We had a rock slide last night."

"A what?"

Her husband, following her in the door, explained that he was in the other room and heard the gallstones hitting the bottom of the toilet bowl as they dropped out. He collected maybe a cup of gallstones that had come out after three days of juice. Instead of $1200 for the operation, it cost them about $12 for the juice and oil. She had no more gallstones, and felt wonderful.

Other herbs used for gallstones are dandelion, golden seal, mistletoe, yellow dock, oak, parsley, and wild yam.

Prevention, however, is the key, and adherence to Dr. Christopher's mucusless diet will prevent the formation of these stones.

CYSTS AND TUMORS

Hundreds of women have wondered why they have tumors and

cysts in their bodies. The cause, according to Dr. Christopher, is potassium deficiency. When a patient takes plenty of potassium foods (not supplements) you can remove the cause of the cysts and tumors. Other foods, which are lower in potassium, must not be increased when you are trying to increase the potassium in the system. When patients go on the three-day cleanse and mucusless diet and take the female corrective and hormone balancing formulas, they receive nourishment which is high in potassium. Miraculous things happen to them. For even faster results, you can add to each cup of herb tea six to ten drops of elderberry tincture or six to ten drops of black walnut tincture, both of which are extremely high in potassium.

Cysts and tumors are like leeches, but they stay in places where there is a body deficiency. As soon as the body is balanced and well, the cysts and tumors have to go, because the material is too healthy for them to live on.

This is why so many patients brought Dr. Christopher cysts and tumors in various sizes that they had expelled from their bodies. There is not enough food, in the form of dying or deficient body materials, so they just decide to leave.

There are several ways to receive your potassium. Dr. Bernard Jensen sells a potassium broth made from dehydrated vegetables. Dr. Bronner makes a similar, excellent product. You can also make your own potassium broth by simmering equal parts of red potatoes, celery, carrots, onions, and herbs to taste. Raw vegetable and fruit juices also flood the system with potassium.

When cysts or tumors grow in places where they can be seen outside the body, often we react by having them cut out. This defeats healing by working on the effect instead of the cause. You can cut cysts out, tumors off, and burn warts off (which are also a potassium deficiency), or get rid of as many moles as you wish, but unless you go to the cause, they will grow back again, and you may end up with as many or more cysts, tumors, moles as before. Different signs of potassium deficiency will keep popping out on the body because the condition that needs correcting is on the inside. You have to go into the cause, Dr. Christopher always insisted, which is the way we have been eating.

Other herbs used for cysts are corn silk, apple cider vinegar, wormwood, cramp bark, chamomile, gravel root, slippery elm, wild carrot, and garlic.

GAS

Some people get gas attacks and it can be very embarrassing, especially in a public place. In Orem, Utah, a lady was having frequent gas attacks. These come mainly because we gulp our food without properly chewing it. She was suffering pains that would cause her to scream. She would call frequently for Dr. Christopher to come and help her. The quickest way he could do so was by reflexology, working on the zones in the feet. She was always very grateful for his help, but always equally embarrassed. As he would work the ascending colon, she would burp and burp, bringing the gas out. But when he would start the transverse colon, then her burps would go to the bottom side, and she would be breaking wind just as fast as he worked her feet. She was really embarrassed. He told her that other people do it too, so not to feel embarrassed.

Some people, he taught, cannot learn to chew their food thoroughly, to eat without gulping. Actually, we can retrain ourselves to eat slowly and to chew, but it might mean breaking a lifetime of bad habits. Aside from reflexology, wild yam tea can help stop those terrible gas pains.

One particular woman was worried that she was dying of a heart attack. Dr. Christopher checked her eyes and told her that there wasn't anything wrong with her heart; in fact, it was in excellent condition. He wished his own heart were as good as hers! He assured her that she was not having a heart attack.

She was somewhat belligerent: "Well, don't tell me, I should know, it's me that's having them. I can be washing dishes and all of a sudden, my heart will stop beating and I fall on the floor and pass out. Or I'll be walking down the street, shopping, and pass out. They rush me to the hospital, and I always come to before anything is done, like operations."

Dr. Christopher told her she hadn't any heart problems at all, but that she did have a condition on her descending colon, where she had a bowel pocket, a gas pocket, and whenever she got gas in that, it pushed up against her heart valves and cut the heart off. That is why the heart would stop, because of the gas pressure. She said that she was having a heart pain right then and that the heart was constantly troubling her. She was afraid she would pass out.

He told her to hang on, and he called on the intercom to the laboratory, where they always had hot water ready. He had them mix up a teaspoon of wild yam and a cup of hot water. Within a very short time he strained out a cup of wild yam tea for the woman. She was just about ready to pass out. She took a couple of drinks of the tea and started to burp. Finally the gas was completely relieved.

After taking Dr. Christopher's advice and not gulping her food, but chewing more thoroughly, using wild yam as she needed, she got over this problem and never had another attack.

Dr. Christopher uses wild yam in his anti-gas formula (see "Formulas" page 202).

Other herbs used for gas are catnip, cloves, garlic, myrrh, pennyroyal, sassafras, spearmint, tansy, thyme, valerian, white poplar, peppermint.

ASTHMA

We mentioned asthma in the section on puberty, but you should know that the drugs doctors prescribe for the condition can be very dangerous. Theophylline is the standard ingredient for most anti-asthmatic medicines, and it has a long list of possible side-effects, including nausea, stimulation of the central nervous system, irritability, sleeplessness and over excitement. We do not know what the long-term effects of the drug might be.

More dangerous still are the steroid drugs, such as Vanceril and Prednisone. If taken by children, these drugs can adversely affect growth and sexual maturation. It encourages yeast infections both locally and systemically. Adrenal insufficiency has been traced to this drug, so severe that death could result. Broken bones become more common among recipients of this kind of drug. When you are ready to take yourself off these drugs, you can suffer all kinds of side effects (withdrawal symptoms), such as inability to maintain body warmth, extreme tiredness, faintness, exhaustion, heart palpitations, and so on.

If you are an asthma sufferer, you should examine the natural way very carefully before exposing yourself to these powerful drugs. A natural source of ephedrine, which is used for congestion, is Brigham tea. This herb, combined with the peppermint/lobelia treatment and an altered lifestyle (including getting rid of problematic tension, which sometimes bring on asthma attacks), can bring you relief safely.

The peppermint/lobelia treatment is well outlined in the following case history taken from the book *Dr. John Raymond Christopher: An Herbal Legacy of Courage;* "One particular patient arrived at the door of Ray's house well past midnight. Ray had just returned to his cozy home from making house calls and was ready to settle wearily beneath the hand-stitched quilts when there came a frantic pounding at the door.

"Pulling his robe over his shoulders, Ray threw open the door. Leaning against the door frame were two young men, each supporting a wizened old man who was struggling for every breath of air. Ray recognized the wheezing sounds of asthma. The man who leaned on the others for support was probably one of the sickest and most pathetic Ray had ever seen.

"Please!' cried one of the young men. 'Our regular doctor is out of town, and we can't find his assistant. Can you help keep Pap alive?' Ray nodded as he ushered the three out of the night air.

"As he settled the gasping old man into a chair and prepared a cup of peppermint tea, Ray listened to the tale of the old man's illness. He had been stricken with asthma for twenty-six years, for twenty of those it had been so severe that he could not hold a job. It had been more than twenty years since he had reclined in bed, for if he lay down, he choked up so severely he risked death. His sons had built him a special chair in which to sleep at night.

"Both sons were working full-time to meet the family's expenses. It wasn't just a matter of keeping a roof over their heads and food on the table, one explained--their father's medical care had devastated their savings and nearly ruined them financially.

"The asthma was now so severe that he required shots, respiratory therapy, and oxygen treatments, often more than twice a week.

"Dr. Christopher knelt by his side and helped him sip the steaming peppermint tea. Ten minutes later, he administered a full teaspoon of tincture of lobelia. Ten minutes later, as the four of them talked, Dr. Christopher spooned in another measure of tincture of lobelia, and ten minutes later, he swallowed the third teaspoonful. Then Dr. Christopher quietly began gathering pots, pans, and buckets.

"Suddenly the man began vomiting. From two until five that morning he threw up, and with it came the thick, stifling, blackened phlegm that had choked his airways. Because he had sipped the cup of peppermint tea, his muscles were relaxed, he suffered no soreness from the hours of heaving.

"Just after five o'clock, well before the morning sun began peeking over the mountainous horizon, Dr. Christopher turned to the boys. 'You can take your father home now; he is finished with the treatment. He is fine now.'

"As the two rushed to their father's aid, he waved them aside with a brush of the hand. 'You don't have to help me, boys,' he said, 'I'll walk.' After seeing them out into the early morning, Dr. Christopher finally settled into bed for an hour's rest before the patients began filling his waiting room again.

"He wasn't the only one who settled into bed that night. As the two young men signaled for their father to sit in his chair, he shook his head. 'Put me to bed, boys,' he insisted. 'I'm going to sleep in a bed tonight.' 'You can't, Pap!' one argued. 'It will kill you!'

"But there was no persuading the man, who was gulping the fresh Evanston air as if it were a feast. He settled into bed and fell into a heavy sleep and slumbered deeply for thirty hours. Finally, he arose from his bed, filled his chest with oxygen for the first time in twenty years, and announced, 'I'm healed. I'm going out to get a job.'

"Years later, a tall, handsome young man stopped Dr. Christopher on the street in Salt Lake City. 'Do you remember the time we woke you in the middle of the night when my dad was having that asthma attack?' Dr. Christopher smiled at the memory. 'Well, it's been years now, and he's never had another attack. He got a job as a gardener, and he's never lost a day's work. He sleeps in a bed every night. We don't know how to thank you. (pages 58-60)"

Besides the lung and respiratory tract formula, and the asthma formula (see "Formulas" page 192 & 200), other herbs which have been used to treat asthma are comfrey, cramp bark, coltsfoot, elecampane, garlic, ginseng, horehound, lemon and honey, licorice root, marshmallow, mullein, mustard, peppermint, pine gum, slippery elm, wild cherry, wintergreen, and yellow dock.

DRUG ABUSE

In 1978, a federal official told a congressional committee that 36 million American women were taking tranquilizers, 16 million were taking sedatives, and 12 million took stimulants, usually diet pills. In 1979, 160 million prescriptions for tranquilizers were filled, but only 10 percent of these were written by psychiatrist, who are the only medical specialists trained to monitor their effects. A federal report related that 60 percent of mind-altering drugs, 71 percent of anti-depressants, and 80 percent of the amphetamines prescribed are given to women. Women are prescribed twice the quantity of drugs as men for the same condition (Mendelsohn, *Male Practice*, p. 60).

Congresswoman Cardiss Collins of Illinois summed it up: "We are all prone to thinking of drug abuse in terms of the male population and illicit drugs such as heroin, cocaine, and marijuana. It may surprise you to learn that a greater problem exists with some 2 million women dependent on legal prescription drugs.

"It is not uncommon for a doctor to advise a male patient to 'work out' his problems in the gym or on the golf course, while a female with the same symptoms is likely to be given a prescription for Valium" (Ibid, p. 61).

Valium, Librium, Placydil--tranquilizers, mood changers--comprise the majority of drugs that women abuse today. This points to one of the main facets of health--mental and emotional contentment. I personally believe that many women are anxious and unhappy at home because in suburban homes or city apartments, we are cut off from each other. In more primitive cultures, people walk outside, work together, talk together, share. This interaction is incredibly healing and productive of joy and contentment. Most women today work and associate in an extremely small circle, often attended with stresses of city life, fast pace, pollution, and general dissatisfaction and imbalance. The happiest and healthiest time I spent was in the Alaskan wilderness, with two or three other families and an assortment of single persons. I was six months pregnant with the biggest baby we've ever had, and I did all my cooking out of doors on a wood fire. We lived in a tent, and ate the simplest of foods. The only entertainment we enjoyed was from books. We rarely set foot inside a building--perhaps we were able to attend church once a month, and sometimes we drove in to shop at a grocery store or visit friends--but mostly we lived quietly and slowly out-of-doors, associating peacefully with one another. Does it sound boring, unproductive, demeaning? Our health improved, our minds worked clearly and effectively, and we were really happy. When we arrived back to our homes in "civilization" we were astonished at the visible tension we saw in others, tension that we soon shared when we started living in that way again.

In addition, Dr. Christopher taught that the desire for stimulants in various forms is caused by malnutrition, improper eating, so that this imbalance attacks the nerve centers of the body and causes cravings. In Evanston, Wyoming, a lady came to see Dr. Christopher for help. She was a registered nurse in the Evanston General Hospital, but she was about to give up. She came to Christopher's as a last resort.

She had started out drinking coffee, and then went on to cigarettes, smoking very heavily. Soon she started to drink. She had become an alcoholic, but alcohol didn't feed the craving she was feeling, so she began taking heavy drugs. She knew that she was fairly well saturated and that it would be hard for her to stop. She had no other way to turn, and was afraid she would lose her job at the hospital because of the bad effects of all these things she'd been taking.

Dr. Christopher told her that the program would not be easy, that it would take time and patience. When he asked her if she would follow it, she said she would do anything they asked her to do.

First, she was to clean her bowels with the lower bowel tonic, and she was very badly constipated. Step two was the red clover combination tea to cleanse her blood stream, to get some of the toxic poisons and wastes from them. Then she was to stick strictly with the three-day cleanse and mucusless diet, going on the three-day cleanse at the beginning of every two weeks. After three months, she reduced the three-day cleanse to once monthly. She was to drink a gallon of steam-distilled water every day, and to stop the use of coffee, tea, tobacco, alcohol, and drugs.

The withdrawal period was very terrible, but she went through it, and at the end of less than a year, she had blossomed out into a different person entirely, a likeable and enjoyable person who could keep her job as long as she liked, because people loved her.

One of the worst side-effects of drug abuse among women is in their children! The little ones watch mother; every time she gets stressed or unhappy, she runs to the cupboard and takes a pill. Children learn much more from example than from preaching, and these will be the young adults who run to drugs to overcome tension and stresses of growing and maturing. When mothers take herb teas, go for walks, visit with neighbors, swim, or eat something wholesome when they get nervous or under stress, the children will do the same. Quite apart from what good we mothers owe ourselves, we owe it to our children to stay strictly away from drugs.

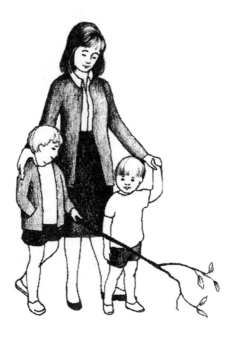

Other herbs used to detoxify drugs from the system are bugleweed, yellow dock, apple pectin, basil and cloves, cayenne, fennel, oatmeal, oat straw, peach pits, alfalfa, clematis, and licorice.

VISION TROUBLES

Dr. Christopher was sitting in his office in Evanston, Wyoming one day, and in walked an elderly, white-haired woman with a little child leading her. The woman was completely blind, and the little child brought her right up to the desk. The woman said she had been blind for over ten years, not able to see anything, using a child or a seeing-eye dog to find her way around. Recently she had heard about Dr. Christopher's eyebright formula and wanted to know if it could help her. Dr. Christopher could not promise her anything, but he said it had done much good and never any harm. He told her about the mucusless diet, because everything works better when you have a cleaner body, and she began the eyewash formula. She kept visiting Dr. Christopher regularly, and he gave her adjustments and other therapies.

One day, she came into the waiting room and into the office, without a seeing eye dog or child. She smiled and said, "Hello Doctor." This was the first time, she said, that she knew what he looked like--just like she had pictured him, she said. She had her eyesight back, truly thrilled, because for ten years she had been walking in a blind world.

"I want to show you how my eyes have healed," she said. She walked over and picked up a book off his desk and read the title on the outside. She opened the book and read several verses.

Dr. Christopher commented that most blind people feel hopeless, but there is hope. Thousands have had their eyesight improved with the eyewash routine, which is one part each bayberry bark, eyebright herb, golden seal root, red raspberry leaves, and 1/8 part cayenne. Make a tea and use as under "Formulas."

When people become blind from cataracts, glaucoma, near- or far-sightedness, there are no two cases alike. Not everyone can be cured, Dr. Christopher stressed. A brother-in-law of his had a torn retina, and the program could not help him at all. Even medical science could do nothing. He had laser beam treatments and other things, without success. But others who have had the same condition have been healed. Some people who have been born blind have been able to see. Two adults and one infant that Dr. Christopher recalls were born blind, and were later able to see, thanks to this program.

If the eye has been damaged by way of chemicals or some other damage, you should know that the eyebright formula was first used to repair an eye injury caused by a batted baseball. With glaucoma or cataracts, though it may take time, there is hope. A lady with cataracts had been blind for a number of years, and yet in nine days she had her full sight back. This astounded Dr. Christopher, for it to have happened so fast. Other people go on the program for as long as three years, and though they then can see better than before, they have not been completely healed. Others clear in a matter of months--it varies with the individual.

Other herbs for treating eye problems include marshmallow, plantain, purple loosestrife, southernwood, wild cherry, rue, chamomile, chickweed, golden seal, squaw vine, red raspberry, tormentil, witch hazel, agrimony, red root, and self heal. Cayenne is also used for eyes, however extreme that might sound. Dr. Christopher recalled a student of his standing in front of a lecture and throwing a pinch of cayenne into one eye. Dr. Christopher was sure the student had lost his senses! But in a few moments the eye stopped watering, and it became clear, bright and healthy-looking.

GANGRENE

Cheryl, a young woman in Yakima, Washington, had lost feeling in her feet. One day she was standing on a floor register and didn't realize how hot it was. She scorched one foot so badly that it had become raw and infected. Gangrene set in and the infection had gone up past her foot and into her ankle, and part way up her knee. She was under the care of the county financially, and when the county agent saw her foot in this gangrenous state he insisted that she go to the hospital and have her leg amputated. At the hospital, all agreed that only amputation could solve the problem; there was no cure for it. She refused, saying she had a friend who could get the gangrene out of her foot. They argued back and forth, and they finally gave her 48 hours to heal the problem.

Jane, one of Dr. Christopher's students, lived in Yakima and knew there was a cure for gangrene. She called Dr. Christopher for help. He gave her step-by-step instructions on what to do. She was to find marshmallow plants, pull them up, and use the entire plant, root to flowers, as a tea. She was to add from a tablespoon to an ounce of cayenne to the tea. In this tea, Jane was to soak Cheryl's leg for thirty minutes, as hot as she could stand it, in a large container so that when the foot was submerged, it could cover the entire place of infection, right up to the knee. After the thirty-minute soak, Jane was to put Cheryl's foot into a container of cold water, as cold as could be taken from the tap, and leave it there for five minutes. This would give Jane time to have ready a new pot of marshmallow tea to soak the foot again. This cycle of 30 minutes tea - five minutes water, was to be repeated throughout the day; a rather strenuous procedure, but necessary in such an extremity. At night, they could put a wet compress on the infection while the girl slept.

The next morning, the whole procedure would be repeated until the infection was clear. In the morning, the pain was already gone. Within forty-eight hours, the gangrene had left the ankle and foot, and there was just a small amount showing in one of the toes. The county agent said to continue with the program and he would keep in touch to see how she was progressing. Cheryl's foot was completely cleared.

Other herbs used for treating gangrene are bayberry, oak, slippery elm, southernwood, beech, beth root, black alder, blackberry, black cohosh, black walnut hulls and leaves, black willow, bladderwrack, blood root, blue violet, burdock, chamomile, cinnamon oil, cloves, comfrey, coriander oil, cranesbill, echinacea, elecampane, elder bark, eucalyptus, fennel oil, sage, garlic, golden seal, holly, horseradish, hydrangea, juniper berry, Irish moss, lemon, lily of the valley, marigold, marshmallow, mullein, myrrh, sanicle, stinging nettle, sumach, thyme, wintergreen, and wood sage.

DIABETES/HYPOGLYCEMIA

Today diabetes is said to be one of the top killers in the world. It is supposedly one of the incurable diseases, but it can be definitely cleared if one approaches it properly. Diabetes stems from a disorder in the pancreas, so you shouldn't just treat it by giving insulin, which is working on the effect; you should instead go to the cause of the disease. Pancreatic malfunction can manifest in one of two ways: diabetes, which is high blood sugar, or hypoglycemia, which is low blood sugar. Though they are completely different, they both stem from the same cause, a malfunction of the pancreas, which is what we have to treat.

Dr. Christopher saw his mother suffer for years from diabetes, and during her life the only treatment was insulin injections, so that his mother's arms, he recalled, looked like pincushions. Although her insulin shots grew progressively more frequent and potent, problems from diabetes continued to trouble her. He watched her die when her diabetes went into Bright's Disease, and then into gangrene, so that she died of gangrene poisoning. At the same time, because of edema, she swelled up to almost half again as big as her normal size. Dr. Christopher, agonizing with her through her pain, prayed that he could find something to help other people so they wouldn't have to suffer as she did.

Later in his practice, Dr. Christopher stumbled onto the herb to heal the pancreas, one which he had never seen in any of his research: the cedar berry herb, *juniperas monostone* berry, that grows on the cedar trees in Nevada, Arizona, and Utah. He learned that these berries not only furnish insulin to the individual, but also heal the pancreas, the main matter of interest in these conditions. Dr. Christopher helped hundreds of people with this, which number grew into thousands when his formulas began selling nationwide.

One day a man and his sister, both middle-aged adults, came into Dr. Christopher's office. She had severe diabetes, and his hypoglycemia was so bad that medical tests indicated that he could not get any worse, and offered no hope to help him. Dr. Christopher told them both to use the mucusless diet and to take the pancreas formula, although they took the lower bowel formula and blood cleansing formula before they began on the pancreas formula.

The woman was using around 80 to 85 units of insulin a day, being a severe case. Despite her initial condition, within a year her pancreas was furnishing its own insulin, and she tapered off gradually until she didn't need it at all. Her brother took a glucose tolerance test in six months and received a clean bill of health; his hypoglycemia was completely cleared.

Despite the fact that they had opposite diseases, diabetes and hypoglycemia, both were cleared because each had a family weakness in the pancreas. When their pancreas was cleared, the diseases were removed.

Sometimes a woman will get hypoglycemia when she conceives or when she undergoes other extreme stress. In addition to the pancreas formula, other treatments can sometimes alleviate the distress. You must realize that the stress might have been experienced sometime in the past, and perhaps a small episode can trigger a hypoglycemic reaction. First of all (and perhaps easier said than done), a woman needs to find ways to reduce the bad affects of the stress. Vigorous exercise out-of-doors, preferably in the country where pollution is minimal, can help you handle stress better. Using low-stress foods, as in the mucusless diet, can give the body stamina to handle situations otherwise overwhelming. Jerusalem artichokes are said to contain insulin, which is a natural substance having some of the effects of insulin. Celery juice is said to be soothing and healing for hypoglycemia --also for diabetes.

Most hypoglycemics have problems feeding themselves, for they crave protein and sugar, yet these substances are wearing on the adrenals, which are often exhausted in hypoglycemics. You need to feed the adrenals with licorice root and hawthorn berries, the latter being said to produce natural adrenalin. You need to take high-quality protein, as in the nuts and seeds and legumes. Sprouted sunflower seeds, sprouted almonds, and chia seeds are all high-quality sources of protein. The other seeds and nuts are good as well. You can soak and low-heat legumes, particularly pinto beans, which are high in potassium and easily digested, for satisfying and long-lasting protein. Be sure that you eat plenty of vegetables, both raw and cooked, in preference to too many fruits, which can overload the system with sugar.

When suffering with hypoglycemia, I devised a power-packed drink which helped every time. In a blender place a handful of soaked or sprouted almonds, a cup or two of water, a banana, some pineapple juice, a tablespoon of brewer's yeast, and a handful of chia seeds. Blend until the seeds thicken the drink. This is mild but very helpful in feeding high-vibration protein to the system.

Other herbs used to treat these conditions are barberry, blue flag, hop tree, marshmarigold, Oregon grape, yellow dock, cranesbill, red raspberry, sumach, and devil's club.

HAIR LOSS

Some people laugh about the loss of hair, although for a woman it can be devastating. Dr. Christopher used to say that the only thing to stop falling hair is the floor--unless you use the right herbs.

He was giving a crash course in herbs to a group of very wealthy women who were going to Europe on a tour. They wanted to know what they could learn about herbs before they left. They were having three lectures a day, four hours per lecture--really a crash course. One of the ladies, an attorney's wife, asked what could be done for the loss of hair. One of the other ladies said, "Let's not waste time on that-- your husband has a good head of hair. There is nothing to worry about."

"Yes, there is something to worry about," the lady responded. "I want to know if a bald-headed person can get his hair back."

"Look," said a third lady, "we are trying to cram this course, and let's get through with it as fast as possible."

None of them thought this lady had any real concern, because she had a beautiful head of hair.

The attorney's wife was crying then, and she jerked off her wig and threw it on the woman's lap, saying that if she liked it so well she could keep it. She was as bald as a cue ball. A hairdresser had used something on her hair, which made it all fall out. So the ladies apologized and wanted to talk about hair loss after all.

Dr. Christopher explained the three-oil massage, which is as follows: The first two days, the patient should be massaged with castor oil, using a clockwise circular motion. This castor oil cleanses and flushes the skin and removes toxins. The second two days, the area is massaged with olive oil, which feeds and rebuilds muscles and flesh. The next two days, wheat germ oil is used for the massage, which heals, being high in vitamin E. On the seventh day the patient rests. Immediately after the massage, the patient takes a sunbath, starting with only two minutes a day and increasing two minutes each day, up to a half hour. Use direct sunlight, though not in the heat of the day, and in cloudy weather use a sunlamp.

The group took off for Europe as planned, and months later Dr. Christopher visited this attorney and his wife on legal matters. The wife's hair was a bit shorter this time, and she said, "Doctor, look at my hair." He thought she had another wig on. "Reach over and pull my hair," she said. Dr. Christopher looked at her husband, who nodded. So he reached over and gave the hair a pull. She said, "Ouch!" She was so delighted that she had a healthy head of hair again. Dr. Christopher had seen this happen many times, including a case where a man was completely bald, who followed the program, and got a full head of hair again--curly this time instead of straight as before!

Other herbs that stimulate the growth of hair are cayenne, birch, dogbane, nettles, red root, and willow.

Yucca root makes up into a lovely natural shampoo.

DEAFNESS, EAR TROUBLES

In many cases, a person can have her hearing restored by following Dr. Christopher's program. One patient had lost her hearing, and could only hear if someone screamed at her when she had her hearing aids turned up full. She couldn't use the phone anymore, and felt discouraged with life in general.

She decided to use the B tincture and garlic oil routine. With an eyedropper, you insert into each ear at night four to six drops of oil of garlic and four to six drops of B tincture, plugging ears overnight with cotton, six days a week, resting on the seventh day. This can continue for four to six months, or as needed. On the seventh day, flush the ears with a small ear syringe using warm apple cider vinegar and distilled water half and half. Be very careful when using a syringe in the ear. Do not release the syringe while inside the ear as this may create a vacuum that can damage the inner ear.

Dr. Christopher commented that many cases where the person was considered legally deaf, by using this program they were able to hear again. Hundreds of people have thrown their hearing aids away after rebuilding their hearing with this simple program.

This same program is used for earaches and roaring in the head, ringing in the ears, etc. Dr. Christopher originally got this formula when he was working with an epileptic. He was searching for something that could really help the case, and received the formula by inspiration, as if a voice were saying it to him. An old gentleman thought that it might help his hearing, so he put it in his ears, too. In that same household, one of the little children had a terrible earache one night. The mother used this combination in the ears, and the pain stopped and the infection cleared up. Many children have been relieved from this simple program of garlic oil and B tincture.

Another special herb used for ear troubles is mullein, made up into oil. We gather the mullein blossoms and steep them in the sun in olive oil for at least three days and up to three weeks. This healing oil is great for any ear problems, as well as being soothing to the entire system. I use it for scrapes and bruises with great success. Chamomile, hops, lobelia, and rue are also used for ear troubles.

PYORRHEA (INFECTION OF THE GUMS)

One night Dr. Christopher decided that he would not give his usual lecture series because there was a blizzard coming on. He figured that nobody would come out on such a night. He was going to put a sign on the door that they would meet the following week. But something said to him, "If you can help just one person, it would be worth staying." So instead of going home, he opened up and put the chairs out. Soon people started coming, and the house was nearly full. He had finished his subject, and said, "We are now going to talk on a subject that has bothered many people, pyorrhea." And just as he began to say this, a woman stepped in the door. The street light showed that the storm was still going, and the woman brushed snow off her coat and stomped it off her overshoes. He said there was another seat available in front, but, crying, she shook her head and stood there by the door.

He continued to tell the audience what to do for pyorrhea, which was to use powdered oak bark, putting it up between the lips and gums at night before going to bed, leaving it in all night. This should be done faithfully six nights a week, week after week. It would tighten the gums and heal, and if the teeth were loose, they would tighten up again. An American Indian remedy, it had cleared many cases of pyorrhea.

As he finished this subject, the door opened and the lady stepped out again. He thought little of it and finished the lecture. But two weeks later during the same lecture series, there was a lady down in front that he didn't recognize. This lady raised her hand and asked if she could say just a few words before starting.

He thought she might be telling about someone who had left their lights on or something, but she stood up and said that she had been at the lecture two weeks before, although no one would recognize her. She was from out-of-town and came in by bus to Salt Lake City. Some time before she had gone to a dentist because her teeth were getting loose. When the dentist looked into her mouth, he said it was the worst case of pyorrhea that he had ever seen in his life. He said that there was nothing that he could do other than to pull all her teeth, trim her gums, and put in a new set of teeth. He didn't feel qualified to do this because he hadn't the equipment or knowledge, but that a specialist in Salt Lake City could do it.

This specialist said he had never seen a case that bad. She had 32 teeth of her own, without a filling, and yet they were all loose; they all had to be pulled. The dentist took an impression of her mouth, and asked her to come back in two weeks, when he would have her false teeth ready and he would pull the teeth and trim the gums.

This nearly broke her heart, because her teeth had been perfect up until then. She went back to her hotel because she couldn't get a bus back home until morning. During the blizzard, she just lay there worrying about losing her teeth and, not being able to rest, got up, dressed, and went out for a walk. She didn't know the town at all, but just walked up one street and down another. She didn't know where she was, and all of a sudden she wound up on State Street right in front of the Christopher store.

The curtain was closed, and a light was shining through it and, feeling chilled, she entered the room just to get warm. Later she felt that the good Lord had her wander around the streets until he knew it was time for Dr. Christopher to talk about pyorrhea. When he finished the subject, she felt that all the weight of the world was suddenly lifted off her shoulders. She knew the right way to be healed. She went right back to her hotel room and slept like a baby. The next day, she found a health store close to the hotel and bought some powdered oak bark. She put it right in her mouth and got on the bus.

Within a matter of days, she went back to her dentist to tell him that her gums were healing and her teeth getting solid again. He had never seen anything like this. He wanted her to go to the specialist in Salt Lake City to show him her mouth. She went to Salt Lake City the day she spoke in the lecture, and the specialist said that in his years of dentistry, he had never seen a miracle like this. He didn't know pyorrhea could ever be healed. He recognized it as an act of God.

She just told the class to listen to what Dr. Christopher told them, because here she stood, with all of her natural teeth intact because of oak bark.

Other herbs used for troubles with teeth and gums include barberry, bistort, cranesbill, oak, Oregon grape, potentilla, self heal, strawberry, and prickly ash. An excellent formula for pyorrhea is the antiseptic tincture. For a toothache, you can use cow parsnip, cranesbill, oak, tobacco and, of course, cloves. Chamomile, cayenne, hops, plantain, prickly ash, and sassafras can relieve pain. Elecampane is said to help with tooth decay.

CONSTIPATION

Dr. Christopher often said there will never be world peace as long as we have a lot of constipated warriors sitting around the peace table. When people are constipated, they are not fit to live around. The nastiest, most antagonistic people you know are apt to be those who are constipated.

One day a lady stomped into Dr. Christopher's office in Evanston, Wyoming. As she came to a screeching halt before his desk, she said she had female problems, and she understood that he had helped other women with female problems. She wanted him to clear her up. She was extremely demanding and abrupt. Because she wore a nurse's uniform from the Evanston General Hospital, he knew she was a registered nurse.

He looked at her and said, "Ma'am, how long since you have had a bowel movement?"

She snapped back at him, "Nine days, so what?"

He apologized about being crude, but he knew that there was something wrong with her. Before they did anything about her female problems, they would have to clear up the bowel area.

She agreed to do anything that he asked her. He told her about the three-day cleanse, mucusless diet, using a gallon of steam-distilled water each day, and to keep her diet as raw as possible. She was also to use the herbal lower bowel formula. He didn't want her to come see him again until she was having three or more bowel movements on her own without using enemas or laxatives. He gave her a large packet of the lower bowel tonic. The average person uses two capsules three times a day, but he told her to use five or more capsules three times a day, and more if needed. He said to keep using them until she got movements. She agreed and left.

This woman had gone from nine to thirteen days between bowel movements for 26 years. That accounted for her being such a nasty individual.

He didn't see her for ten days, and when she came in, instead of stomping in and growling at him, she glided in and said, "Oh, good morning, isn't it a beautiful morning?"

"You must have been using the lower bowel tonic."

She said that she had, and that it was working.

"How many did you have to use to get started?"

"I had to use forty to forty-five capsules a day before I broke loose, and now I am down to five or more three times a day."

In a month, she was down to two capsules three times a day. At the end of a year, she was having three or more bowel movements a day without using any bowel tonic at all. The lower bowel tonic is not a habit-forming laxative; it is a food. It rebuilds the peristaltic muscle in the bowel, and gets it working again, and also cleans up the liver and gall bladder. It changed her whole life.

At the end of the year, she was moving her bowels regularly and easily, with no aids at all except the foods, which were of a mucusless type. She was a different woman entirely. In fact, she was so changed that other nurses and interns came to get the lower bowel capsules from Dr. Christopher, because they said anything that could change that woman's horrible disposition must be a good thing.

So many herbs are used for constipation that it is hard to enumerate them all. They include almonds, apples, apricots, carob, cascara sagrada (small), chicory, dandelion, elder flowers and berries, fennel, figs, flaxseed, licorice, marshmallow, motherwort, mountain flax, mustard, oats, olive oil, Oregon grape, Orsa clay, parsley, peach, prickly ash berries, prunes, raspberries, salsify, senna pods, sesame, slippery elm, spinach, strawberry, turkey rhubarb, watermelon, wood betony.

OVERWEIGHT

A woman came to see Dr. Christopher in despair; she said her husband was about to leave her. She now wore a size eighteen dress, but when they had married she wore a size thirteen. She was so fat that her husband became disgusted, she said. Love had flown out the window.

Dr. Christopher simply put her on the mucusless diet and the three-day cleanse. He told her it was not a crash diet, but that she would go down a dress size every few months.

She was faithful to the program because she loved her husband and wanted to keep their family--with children--intact. She came down to her size thirteen and her husband bought her a complete new wardrobe, he was so pleased. She was one of the happiest women Dr. Christopher had ever seen and she invited Dr. Christopher and his family over for dinner.

It was a real vegetarian spread, but the most touching part of it came after dinner. They said, "We are going to have a little ceremony out in the back yard." So out they went, children and all, and there was a grave dug, with some wildflowers on the mound. They asked the Christopher's to sit in chairs there. The children were told to go and prepare the funeral.

Dr. Christopher thought maybe one of their pets had died. But the children came out of the house carrying, each of them, pots and pans that were very expensive aluminum ware--the most expensive you can buy--and put those pots and pans into the grave. Without saying a word, they went to their outside fruit cellar, and brought out slabs of bacon and old hams that were down there, and buried them with the pots and pans. The Christopher's could hardly suppress their feelings.

It was especially touching, because this was during the post-war years when foods were still scarce, so it was quite a sacrifice to bury these items.

Best of all, the wife felt like a new woman, and her husband was very much in love with her again.

We were travelling once, accompanied by a young woman who was somewhat overweight. Just by eating our simple diet, she suddenly began to lose weight. She was astounded that it could happen in such a short time, a period of weeks, and without pain.

A diet of vegetables and fruits, nuts and seeds, and especially the complex carbohydrates--whole grains--will make one lose weight steadily. You won't experience a dramatically quick loss, as with high-protein diets. High protein diets can be dangerous. They build the toxin level in the body, and they turn up your "fat thermostat," which means that your body receives messages that it's starving, and you feel tremendously hungry so that you eat until the fat comes back on again. You can end up heavier in the long run.

If you combine the mucusless diet with a consistent exercise program, you will lose the weight and keep it off. As long as you comply with this diet, you can literally stuff yourself and you won't gain weight.

The kind of exercise required for this diet should be aerobic, which means that it raises the rapidity of the heartbeat for a period of time, at least a half hour preferably. Aerobic exercise includes fast walking, jogging, swimming (excellent), bicycling, horseback riding, and so on. It also includes dancing, which is what most people think of when they hear the term "aerobics." But you should be careful to stay away from hard rock or similar music, which can be distressing to the system. Some research has indicated that the rock beat stresses the body because it is directly contrary to the heartbeat. One study placed plants in two identical growing rooms; in one room, rock music played constantly, and in the other classical music played. After a period of time, the plants in the rock room shriveled and died; they grew as far away from the source of the music that they could. On the other hand, the plants in the classical room grew *towards* the music, and they thrived. The music you exercise to can really affect your body as well as your mind.

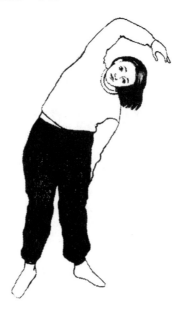

Which brings us to a central point--if you want to lose weight, you need to heal your *mind* of overweight as well as your body. Many of us hold onto weight because we are holding onto negative feelings--grudges, hurts, and so on--that keep us feeling negative. Through meditation or prayer we can work out some of these problems and let them go, and then letting the weight go will even be easier.

Other herbs employed in losing weight include a monodiet of the healing vegetables, such as carrots or cabbage, and spirulina. Other seaweeds can feed the body to overcome imbalance. Chickweed can also help to reduce body fat by suppressing appetite.

OSTEOPOROSIS

Currently of intense interest, osteoporosis is supposedly treated by taking extra calcium. When a woman with osteoporosis has a blood test, the calcium level is usually not low. But in order to be assimilated, calcium must be present in the body with the appropriate synergistic minerals, in particular phosphorus, which must be approximately twice the amount of calcium, and also silica. Without these minerals, and probably other trace minerals that haven't been linked to the problem yet, the body cannot absorb calcium; it just flows through the body, sometimes depositing and causing gout, arthritis, etc. The amount of calcium in the body doesn't matter; it's the balance you take in foods that's important.

For example, when people have broken bones, if their blood calcium is high and their silica low, the bones heal slowly, but if it's the opposite--with low calcium and high silica--the bones heal rapidly.

Usually the right foods will provide the correct mineral balance that will naturally avoid osteoporosis. The calcium formula as well as the bone, flesh, and cartilage formula can provide concentrated sources of minerals for those who are chronically deficient.

When my fingernails have become soft in the past, I have taken calcium supplements in order to harden them, without very good results. But when I am eating many raw, leafy greens, the high concentration of proper minerals harden the nails right up.

Sometimes the imbalance in the system can be brought on by hormonal imbalances, so the hormone-estrogen formula can effectively balance the hormone system.

If your diet is adequate and you are still out of balance, it may be that you are not digesting your food properly; this especially occurs later in life, when the body doesn't produce adequate hydrochloric acid for digestion. The apple cider vinegar and honey mixture--a tablespoon of vinegar and a teaspoon of honey mixed well into a cup of distilled water--taken three times a day, can correct a hydrochloric acid deficiency.

Your intestinal flora may need replacing, which can also cause imbalance in the system. However, taking yogurt probably will not do the job, because most yogurt consists of only one strain of bacteria which, while useful, might not be the one that you need. A multi-strain acidophilus is better. Even cheaper than that is Rejuvelac, which is made by soaking one cup of wheat--previously washed--for forty-eight hours in three cups of water. Use the same seed to make a second and third batch, not rinsing the seed in between. These batches need soak only twenty-four hours. This Rejuvelac, as you can see, is really cheap, and yet provides the ferments which can help restore proper intestinal flora.

If your pancreas is inhibiting digestion, you can add the herbal pancreas formula to your healing routine. For more details about this formula, see section on "Diabetes/Hypoglycemia", on page 132.

REFLEXOLOGY

You can learn what's ailing you by going the medical route, by visiting a chiropractor, or by testing through kinesiology. But the easiest, and cheapest methods of diagnosing non-emergency conditions might be iridology and reflexology. Iridology does require some expertise to perform correctly; with a chart of the iris marked with the various areas of the body, you compare the person's iris and locate problem areas.

Reflexology, on the other hand, is easier to do and very accurate. Obtain a good reflexology chart, usually available through health food stores, and begin to press the areas on the bottom of the foot. Anywhere you locate a sore spot, look it up on your chart to see what it is. For example, if the pancreas spot keeps turning up sore, and you have experienced some symptoms of hypoglycemia, you can assume your pancreas needs treating. If your descending colon is sore, you are likely congested--constipated--and need the lower bowel tonic. I have seen this work remarkably well with people from infants through old age. One elderly lady couldn't figure out exactly what was wrong with her. As I worked her feet, the stomach area kept presenting soreness. So I told her it was probably her stomach, although she denied any problems in that area. Finally her discomfort got so bad that she went to the doctor. What did he diagnose? It was her stomach!

You can also help treat ailments by working those sore spots until they lose their soreness. Reflexology is simple, inexpensive, accessible to the layman, and it works.

HEADACHES

Headaches can stem from several sources. Very common is the constipation headache, where compressed fecal matter presses on the nerves that affect the head. We have seen severe migraine headaches cured by taking a catnip enema. For longer-term relief, the lower bowel formula can heal the bowel so that there is no constipation.

Food allergies are another very common cause of headache. The worst culprit is sugar; I have experienced sugar headaches, which are sort of a withdrawal; you eat the sugar, and then as the body is trying to eliminate the toxic substance, your head pounds. Cheese commonly causes headaches, probably the worst of the dairy products for this, although allergies to any of them may cause the pain. Meats and eggs are also common allergens.

As for other foods, Dr. Christopher used to say that no wholesome food causes an allergic reaction, and if we seem to be allergic to citrus, corn, wheat or whatever, it may be because we have toxins in our systems that react with the foods, for which the cure is the elimination diet. It also may be that we are not chewing our foods properly; the undigested particles irritate the system and cause an allergy-like reaction. The easiest way to check if we are experiencing allergy headaches is to go on the three-day cleanse. Then add one food at a time, and when you get the allergic reaction, you can know you're allergic to that food.

Stress brings on many headaches in women. When we cannot deal with the feelings we have, our heads can pound. Before trying to deal with the deeper issues, there are some remedies that we can apply for immediate relief. Often our bodies are depleted and need immediate nourishment. My favorite headache/stress remedy is blending a banana into a cup of pineapple juice, adding a bit of nutmilk, and mixing in one to two tablespoons of brewer's yeast, blending briefly. In fifteen minutes I am calm and ready to deal with the problems that cause the stress.

Peppermint tea is an old favorite for dealing with headache. Sweeten it with honey if desired. Chamomile, thyme, and ginger tea are traditional too. You can put ginger into a bath and soak to eliminate the tension and pain. Rub your feet against the tap for a crude but effective reflexology treatment. Valerian tea is a sedative and pain reliever.

A thorough reflexology treatment on the feet, working out sore spots as much as possible, can be a good remedy for a headache if the body is in decent shape. Recently I worked on a woman's feet with so many sore spots that she thought I was sadistically pressing hard. She needed a complete cleanse before the accupressure would relieve the terrible headaches she suffered.

For a really severe migraine headache, apply cold packs to the neck and head while the patient soaks in a very hot tub or whirlpool. Be sure to drink lots of feverfew tea and water, take copious amounts of calcium formula and try to enjoy the bath. Apply Professor Cayenne's

Deep Heating Balm, which is an all natural cayenne ointment, to neck and shoulders and give a thorough massage. This relieves many severe headaches, including migraines.

Sometimes people get headaches because they are dehydrated. You would be surprised that most people walk around in a state of dehydration. You need about a gallon of steam-distilled water each day in order to stay completely hydrated.

A good overall body massage, working the muscles to put more energy in when the muscles are strained, can relieve the tension enough to get rid of a headache. Use olive oil or another high-vibration oil to lubricate the skin.

My husband gets severe migraines occasionally, presumably because he does high-stress academic work. These headaches can keep him sitting up all night because they hurt too much for him to lie down. Once when he was suffering from one of these I thoroughly rubbed his back with Deep Heating Balm rubbing out the tense places as much as I could. Soon he was asleep and slept all night.

You can do physical therapy with a person, adjusting or moving him until he reaches a point where it doesn't hurt, and holding that until he is released.

Be sure that you get regular outdoor exercise. Sometimes people exercise and then stop, so the toxins build up in their bodies and cause headaches. Just being outdoors and moving vigorously can clear up a headache.

It may take some time meditating, praying, and talking with the people involved to work out the causes of stress, but if you combine prayer with action you will be surprised how problems can really be solved. If your body and mind are clear enough to work through the conflicts, you will be able to handle them.

Other herbs used to treat headaches are birch, clematis, false Solomon's seal, pennyroyal, poplar, self heal, willow, valerian, lady's slipper, wild lettuce, balm of gilead.

EMOTIONAL HEALTH

I believe that it is harder to live normally and happily today than it has ever been before. Even such elemental topics as food and family become complex and a matter for disputation and experiment. So many of us live in cities or suburbs where the air and land have lost much of their natural vitality because of pollution.

So many women turn to drugs--especially tranquilizers--to relieve the emotional stresses that they feel (see section on "Drug Abuse", on page 126). Unfortunately, these tranquilizers can contribute to the problems they purport to solve. Specifically, tranquilizers interfere with the natural cycles of sleep. The most healing comes during the Rapid Eye Movement sleep (REM), the dreaming time, not the deep sleep that precedes it. However, tranquilizers keep you in the deep sleep stage and don't allow for the lighter REM sleep. Therefore, you can't rest out and your sleep is not healing. REM sleep brings dreams, which are healing and important to mental health; in many traditional cultures, people discuss their dreams in their family groups as a way of understanding themselves in relation to the world and universe. Religions often point to dreams as sources of divine knowledge. By cutting ourselves off from this important source of self-realization, we really inhibit solving the problems we grapple with.

Curiously, certain foods dramatically increase some people's anxieties. Chemical additives, whether preservatives, colors, or enhancers, can make us feel edgy and not ourselves. Sugar hypes us up and lets us down so we feel depressed. Heavy proteins can give us a feeling of dragginess and inability to work. Almost any processed food tends to make us feel as though our teeth are on edge, and it takes at least three days to eliminate the bad effects of some non-food we have taken into our systems.

It may sound too simplistic, but just give it a try and see the difference. A wholesome diet of simple foods can give us tremendous emotional stability. You can add Dr. Christopher's nerve herbal food formula if you need to heal and soothe the nervous system further. It feeds the nerves and heals frayed nerve sheaths. Celery juice and plenty of lettuce in salad can help relax you.

Even our clothing affects our emotions. Dr. Christopher assured us that natural fibers worked in harmony with our bodies, while synthetics have vibrations that work against the human vibration. Years ago when I used to wear synthetics, I would often feel jumpy, irritable, and as if I wanted to jump out of my skin. When I began wearing cottons, wools, and silks--and there are other good natural fibers--much of this nervousness disappeared. In addition, natural fibers allow our skin to breathe and give off toxins. As a matter of interest, rayon is made out of cellulose; it is sometimes called the "natural synthetic." It's the only man-made fiber that comes close to behaving like a natural.

Exercise can help us work out emotional problems. Sometimes medical doctors encourage people--usually men--to work out their pent-up frustrations on the golf course or basketball court. Women, of course, need strong exercise as well. Often our bodies are begging for it, crying out for a good workout. We live in the rolling foothills, and sometimes when I am ready to burst with the day's demands, a fast walk up and down the steep hills will drain away the negative forces so that I can cope.

Still, you need to fix your head as you fix your body. But that doesn't always mean professional help. Research shows that psychological therapy has had a negative effect on people counselled. For example, antisocial and criminal behavior were highest among men who received one-on-one counseling when they were boys. Psychologists counsel people more by apparent factors (finances, political views, or even the ability to hire a lawyer when psychological issues were considered in the courtroom) rather than personality factors. Often counseling of couples experiencing marital problems results in divorce. And most people undergoing standard psychological counseling come out more unhappy than they were when they started (for the research supporting these contentions and a more expanded discussion of this controversial issue, see *The People's Doctor*, Vol. 2, No. 10).

Far better equipped to discuss emotional problems are those who care about us: family, friends, religious leaders. These people want us to succeed in solving our conflicts; they do not take an unattached view guided by textbook principles. This is not to discount the credibility of all counselors, but usually the standard psychiatrist's office is not the place to overcome emotional difficulties.

We need to learn to stand and cope with our problems instead of running from them. Researchers at BYU are probing the logical idea that our conscious choices determine what we do, not our babyhood or any other unconscious condition. Failure to take this responsibility results in self-deception, which seems to be almost a national condition. Most of us refuse to take responsibility for what we are, and yet doing so doesn't hurt us, but only grows us more mature. People practicing meditation and a spiritual approach to life say the same thing; as one mother put it, struggling with acceptance that her baby had died in utero, said, "I'd never seen before what a free-will decision it is to be crazy" (Ina May Gaskin, *Spiritual Midwifery*, p. 451).

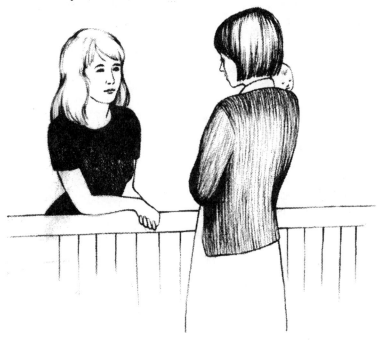

One of our dear friends, an adopted grandfather, suggested that we can struggle with our problems, think them through, work out several solutions, but not come to any resolution. Then we go to sleep, and during our sleep, we may have a dream, or simply allow our unconscious mind to work through the problem, and in the morning we often have the solution or the best course to begin to take.

To heal very difficult emotional problems, resulting from abuse or other violations, we may require help. But standard psychoanalysis may not do it. If you are open and searching, I believe that help, in the form of an appropriate therapy or person, will come to you. I am also certain, because of personal experience, that if we act and reason with integrity, and pray with humility, the answers will come to us beyond our own power to bring them. Experiencing this develops the faith to continue to look to God for answers to our often very complex problems.

INSOMNIA

Dr. Christopher told the story of a high school teacher who had a terrible case of insomnia. She could only sleep in twenty-minute stretches; thereafter, she would pace the floor throughout the night, keeping her family awake and becoming more and more tired herself. During the day she epitomized the "witch" school teacher. Eventually her screaming and irritability, her meanness and nagging, became so intolerable that her family wanted to have her committed to a mental institution. And she was so weary of it all that she would have liked to go herself.

The family called Dr. Christopher, however, who came over and prepared a cup of his nerve herbal food formula tea. As it steeped, he chatted with the family, and then she drank the cup. Soon she yawned and said she might like to go lie down. Her husband commented that Dr. Christopher might just as well stay, because she would be up again in twenty-minutes, but Dr. Christopher took his leave.

The next morning, Dr. Christopher answered the telephone; a man's voice began berating him and calling him all sorts of vulgar names. "You ought to be jailed," the man shouted, "for giving my wife heavy drugs when you said they were herbs!"

Dr. Christopher explained he had only given the woman herbs, so mild that a newborn baby could safely use them. When the man calmed down, he explained that his wife had slept all night, and awakened calm and refreshed.

She continued taking this formula, and cleaned up her diet as well. Before long, she was as sweet and cooperative as she could be with her family and her classes, and everyone was grateful that she didn't have to be committed to a mental institution!

Some other techniques can help you get to sleep. Very effective is the combination of bath and massage, particularly with a soothing oil, such as chamomile. Herbal oils are easily made; see the chapter "Preparations," on page 205. Chamomile and linden tea both can help a person relax and sleep. For a really stubborn case, take a cup of valerian tea or a couple of capsules with warm water.

A pleasant walk out of doors can help a person relax enough to sleep. Sometimes the person's blood sugar is a little low, and simply eating a piece of fresh fruit can put a person out. Warm tea with honey will do the same.

Jean Liedloff describes the Yequena Indians as regarding sleeping and wakefulness as equally desirable. Sometimes the Indians would waken in the night and tell a joke, whereupon everyone would laugh, and all would go back to sleep. Perhaps in our culture we place too much emphasis on the process of getting to sleep. With exercise, fruitful work, and a good diet, getting to sleep might not be so difficult if we change our mental set about it. You can always use Mary Poppins' technique who sang a sleepy lullaby, "Stay awake; don't go to sleep..."

PMS

PMS is easily treated by the natural routine. It doesn't disappear overnight, but with persistence you will notice suddenly that it's gone.

You need to be sure that your bowels are moving properly. Dr. Christopher defined this as three or more bowel movements per day. So often our female problems are directly related to constipation, toxins we are absorbing from our colons. The lower bowel formula and the mucusless diet easily correct constipation.

In addition, you can take the female corrective formula and the hormone balancing formulas to work out problems in the feminine tract. These formulas can correct almost any problem you might have; they are non-specific and they are mild, so you can take them over a prolonged period of time without any problems.

If you exercise well in addition to following the above suggestions, eventually your PMS should disappear. For coping with the problem while you are healing, hot peppermint, catnip or chamomile tea can relieve some of the pressure; try Dr. Christopher's nerve herbal food formula. Good foods containing vitamin-B, such as sprouted wheat and brewer's yeast, and those containing vitamin-C, such as lemons and rose hips, are excellent for balancing the system.

If your PMS is related to emotional issues related to womanhood or relationships, by patient searching you may be able to find the person or therapy you need to help you overcome it. An herbalist asked me, "You're on a healthy program. Do you get PMS?" I admitted that I didn't (although I nurse my babies so long that I don't often have to face the problem). He said that his wife didn't get PMS either, and I have noticed that women who follow the mucusless diet and who exercise eventually find they aren't struggling with the problem anymore. As simple as it sounds, the program works.

YEAST INFECTION

It almost seems that there is an epidemic of yeast infection around the country. Almost everywhere, women ask me what I suggest for candidias albicans, and many feel that their health is truly compromised by it. Basically, a yeast infection occurs when the yeasts, which are naturally present in our bodies, and indeed everywhere in the air, grow out of control in the body. Such a variety of symptoms result that it is hard to pinpoint them, but basically weariness, craving for sweets, irritability, hunger for sweets and starches after a full meal, frequent infections, etc., seem to point to a yeast infection.

I wonder if we are prone to yeast infections because our lives are so out of harmony. One doctor has suspected that emotional patterns and stress generally predispose us to yeast infection. Certainly our diets contain unbalancing factors heretofore unknown; never before has man downed as many chemicals as he is doing today, and who knows how long they might linger in the body?

Basically, the long-term treatment sounds simplistic, but I believe it works: The mucusless diet, emphasizing raw things but not excluding cooked, using live grains instead of flour products, and cleansing the system with the lower bowel tonic and red clover combination when that seems necessary. One health food store worker said that it's easy to overcome yeast infection: Just starve it out--no fruits, no sweets, no grains. But that seems to me defeating. The mucusless diet is satisfying and delicious, and you don't have to eliminate all those things. Certain herbs are antifungal, such as garlic, cayenne, pau d'arco, and black walnut.

While you're in the process of gradually reducing the yeast population in your body, several approaches can help you deal with the symptoms. First follow the slant board routine (see index). Other aids include taking internally a multi-strain acidophilus regularly, and if the yeast infects the vagina, you can insert an acidophilus capsule or two right inside the vagina. Take certain foods that inhibit yeast growth, including olive oil, onions, garlic (raw for medicinal effect or in capsules), cayenne. Avoid yeast-conducive foods, including yeast breads, sugars, concentrated sweets, and anything that contains mold, either intentionally, such as cultured cheeses, fermented drinks, etc., or unintentionally, such as fruits left to go slightly bad. Golden seal, garlic, or apple cider vinegar can be used as a douche if you are not pregnant, and if the yeast is causing vaginal irritation. Wear only cotton underwear, or go without underwear. Don't wear tight pants which cut off the air from the area.

Internally, you can take echinacea tincture, which works wonderfully on any kind of infection. You might also try to find homeopathic Candida Albicans which can quickly help relieve your condition.

Accupressure treatments and stress reduction techniques, including plenty of outdoor exercise, can contribute to your overall anti-yeast program.

When we lived three months outdoors in Alaska, eating very simple foods, never sleeping indoors and rarely going inside a building or a car, we were astonished to find our yeast symptoms virtually disappearing. I think that the sun, air, and pure water might be the best cures for yeast infection, along with a proper diet.

TECHNOLOGY

Most of us accept high technology as a proper fact of life, while mankind has survived in health without these practices for thousands of years. Although the issue is extremely controversial, I believe that certain technologies can be dangerous to our health.

For example, although dentists and doctors assure us otherwise, some scientists assert that routine X-ray techniques can endanger our health. They say that dental X-rays as usually administered "without question increase the significance of a number of central nervous system disorders, tumors, thyroid cancers, and leukemias among our population" (*The People's Doctor*, Vol. 2, No. 5, p. 1). Thyroid cancer has developed from as little radiation as is produced by 10 bite-wing dental X-rays, and a single abdominal X-ray of a pregnant woman can predispose the child to leukemia. Some say that our lifespan is shortened by the aging effects of radiation. Diabetes, cardiovascular disease, stroke, high blood pressure and cataracts have also been associated with radiation effects. Some experts link the incidence of birth defects among older pregnant women (above 35 supposedly being high-risk) is not because the mother is older but because of the accumulation of radiation in the mother's system.

The easiest approach to X-rays is to refuse them categorically except in accidents and threatening situations, such as when our five-week-old Sarah had pneumonia and the doctors needed to know the exact condition of her lungs. Even then, I consented with reservations, but we need to accept the few cases where medical intervention is necessary.

I always wondered why I felt dizzy, nauseous, and unfocused whenever I faced a computer terminal. I used to think that I had a touch of flu, was stressed, overtired, or something. But recent research is linking health problems to video display terminals, the screens on which computer information is presented. Although the technology is far too new to have controlled research conducted on it, clusters of women who use certain VDT's have experienced unprecedented miscarriages and birth defects. There is no movement to test radiation emissions from VDT's, and it can vary dramatically from machine to machine. In addition, prolonged use of computers can cause eyestrain, stress and perhaps some biological effects from positively charged ions (*Mothering*, Spring 1986, pp. 68-77).

John Ott, the pioneer in researching the effects of light on humans (he has shown that living organisms require full-spectrum light for full health; standard light bulbs can reduce health and fluorescent lights are really threatening), did some experiments with VDT emissions. He placed bean plants about ten feet away from a VDT that had leaded glass on it, and protected them with three solid lead shields between. This plant suffered from mottling and yellowing of the leaves, which eventually just dropped off. He removed the plants into a standard greenhouse, which restored them to health, but when he put them back in front of the VDT, they got sick again. In addition, working with a local chiropractor, they placed a drop of human blood on an ultraviolet-transmitting microscope slide, covered with a standard cover slip, and propped it up against a VDT. In five minutes, the red blood cells began to clump into long chains called rouleaux, which can clog the capillaries and cut down blood supply to the brain, possibly contributing to such conditions as Alzheimer's disease. When the blood sample was placed in full-spectrum light, the rouleaux broke apart and the blood resumed normalcy. They also tested the blood of a friend, who is a real computer buff, and found that after an eight-hour day in front of the computer, his blood showed severe rouleaux clumping. After a weekend of full-spectrum light, his blood tested normal again. Apparently lead shielding on computers has no effect at all, although shielding on television screens seems to reduce the bad effects of that radiation (*Mother Earth News*, January/February 1986, pp. 21-22). John Ott has published several books on the subject of light, radiation and health; you can order them from the Downtown Bookshop, 1500 Main St., Sarasota, FL 33577. Both from our intuitive feelings and from this kind of research, we completely avoid computers, television and video showings. This very controversial stand is beginning to be proven scientifically, and we expect that one day it will be indisputable. See our chapter on "Pregnancy," page 32 for information on ultrasound danger.

URINARY INFECTION

As one who has suffered a severe urinary tract infection, I assure you that when it is full-blown, it is a very distressing disease. I could hardly walk when I went to the doctor and, for one of the few times in my life, received antibiotic treatment.

You can treat a urinary infection before it becomes too severe. The best infection fighters--garlic and echinacea--can be started immediately. You would be sure to drink plenty, as the fluid will wash the infection from the system. Hot lemon juice and water, lightly sweetened with maple syrup, is a pleasant healer. You can take cranberry juice, as it is a traditional treatment for the problem, but grocery store cranberry juice is loaded with corn syrup, which is really a source of sugar. Unsweetened cranberry juice is sour. You can make your own by blending some fresh or frozen cranberries with water and straining.

Uva ursi, yarrow, juniper berries and horsetail grass can also help clear up a urinary infection.
To prevent infection, wipe from front to back after using the bathroom, be sure that you and your husband are clean prior to intercourse, and wear cotton underwear or no underwear at all.

Mono diets and any poor foods that unbalance the body's acidity can cause urinary tract infections. Eating excessive amounts of a single type of food such as citrus, potatoes, lima beans, soybeans, beet greens, parsnips, spinach, dried vegetables, cantaloupe, dried fruits, molasses, almonds, chestnuts, and coconut can unbalance the acidity of the body making it more susceptible to infection. A wholesome diet, according to Dr. Christopher means eating a wholesome balance of the wholesome foods found in your area. Milk, sugar, refined flour and soda pop in any amount can adversely affect the acid balance of the body.

You should also avoid chemicals--such as bubble bath--while bathing, and scrub the tub with baking soda.

HEART DISEASE

Heart problems can stem from many sources, too many to go into here. The important thing is to minimize medical intervention as much as possible, because the drugs given for heart problems can often cause side-effects as bad as the heart disease itself.

Dr. Christopher found that hawthorn berries, garlic, and wheat germ oil specifically strengthen the heart. Cayenne has saved lives when a person has suffered heart attack; a teaspoonful in a cup of warm water has equalized the blood pressure and stopped the heart attack. Lecithin helps break down cholesterol, as does natural-source vitamin C.

You should be sure to avoid alcohol, tobacco, and refined foods completely; stay on the mucusless diet, and exercise consistently and moderately in appropriate ways for your condition.

Reflexology can help restore heart health over the long-term. A natural practitioner can often help in a heart attack or restore heart rhythm by using massage and accupressure techniques.

Other herbs said to support the heart and circulatory system are angelica, ginger, golden seal, vervain, licorice root, blue cohosh, peppermint, wintergreen, wood betony, mistletoe, coriander, valerian, blessed thistle, ginseng, and red raspberry leaves.

ALLERGIES

Dr. Christopher used to say that there is no such thing as an allergy to good wholesome food. It if is organic and has no chemicals added, if it is fresh, you should experience no allergic symptoms--that is, if you are digesting your food. You can take the combination of one tablespoon apple cider vinegar and one teaspoon honey in a cup of distilled water before meals to help with the hydrochloric acid in your stomach. If candidias albicans is preventing good digestion, check our section on "Yeast Infection," on page 152. Be sure that you chew all your food thoroughly, including swishing juices around in the mouth to initiate digestion.

The herbal pancreas formula and liver and gall bladder combination can help these organs do their proper job in digestion.

You may be a hayfever sufferer. Pollen triggers an immune-system reaction and throws the body into an elimination cycle. For symptomatic relief, you can take local pollen to clear it up. Don't take massive doses, though; 1 grain at a time is all you need to get started, building up gradually as you can. The allergies, sinus, and hayfever formula, contains herbs which work immediately on the problem, such as Brigham tea, being an antihistamine, and those that clean up the system generally for permanent relief. You can also take the sinus congestion formula (Ephedratean), which includes cayenne and horseradish, for powerful, immediate relief.

If your body is loaded with toxins, your hayfever symptoms might be more severe. Sometimes people react violently to chemicals, perfumes, exhausts, etc. You can do as we do, and try to avoid these substances as much as practical. The cleansing program should help desensitize your body to these allergens.

FIRST AID

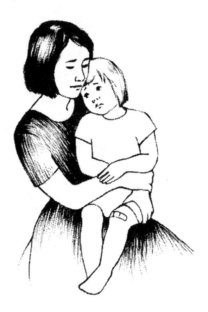

"Mother!" is the first call when someone gets hurt, and so it's good to know a little herbal first aid.

You'll most commonly have to treat skin wounds of various kinds. Usually all you need to do is wash the wound well with soap and water, pat it dry with clean gauze or a clean cloth, and treat it with a good herbal ointment. Because of the combination of antiseptic and soothing qualities, comfrey/marshmallow/marigold ointment is very good. For wounds with the chance of infection, apply X-ceptic, an herbal antiseptic, or marigold tincture. Garlic juice or onion juice kill germs, as does cayenne (stings!). Mullein ointment, comfrey ointment, or other similar soothing herbal ointments are wonderful.

Abscessed Tooth. See your dentist. An old and effective treatment for abscess is tincture of myrrh, applied frequently on the gums. This tincture is also good for mouth irritations generally. Lobelia is also good for abscess.

Appendicitis. This condition generally could not happen if we were not constipated. Mucus forming foods can also bring it on. Take a hot herb enema of spearmint, catnip, white oak bark, bayberry bark, or wild alum root. Plain water may also be used if necessary. Catnip enemas will relieve the pain. Apply hot and cold fomentations to the appendix area and the full length of the spine. At night, apply a poultice of mullein and lobelia, sprinkling with ginger or cayenne. Mix the dried and ground herbs with boiling water to make a paste, thickening with slippery elm or cornmeal. Apply as warm as the patient can stand, leave until cool, then repeat. Use reflexology on the appropriate areas of the feet.

Go on a liquid diet, using fruit juices, potassium broth, and slippery elm gruel. Watch the symptoms closely. This approach should relieve them, but if not, be sure to see a physician.

Bruises. Apply a fomentation of wheat grass juice. Apply the burn paste. Apply a comfrey poultice. These are superior treatments, but other herbs, such as cayenne, chaparral, marshmallow, mullein, myrrh, pennyroyal, rue, and slippery elm can treat bruises as well.

For **burns and deep cuts,** you may wish to check with a physician if you suspect that the nerves or some other vital connection are damaged. One family considered their son's cut deep but not too serious. Checking with a doctor, however, they found that he had severed a complex of nerves, requiring three days of microsurgery! Cleanse the wound and use Dr. Christopher's burn ointment, which is made by blending equal parts of wheat germ oil and honey in a blender, and adding comfrey leaves, fresh or dried, until the mixture becomes thick. I sometimes add a little slippery elm. This mixture is fantastic. It keeps the wound moist but helps restore flesh to its proper condition. Two boys were playing with gasoline, and an explosion burned both of their hands terribly. One of them was taken for standard medical treatment, with the result that his hands healed up like two claws for the rest of his life. The parents of the other child took him to Dr. Christopher, who applied the above burn ointment. The parents were not to remove the dressing, but just add more and more on top of the original.

The boy's hands healed perfectly, with just a little scarring to remind the family of the danger of playing with fire!

One of our children jumped off a table and landed wrong on a foot, breaking one of the bones. We didn't realize the bone was broken until a couple of days later. The usual medical treatment would be to rebreak the bone, set it, and put it in a cast.

Instead, for a week, during the night, we plastered burn ointment all over the foot, bound it up in a white strip of cloth, and pinned a washcloth around that. Within a week that foot was completely healed, the bone set properly, and the child could run and play as before.

Dr. Christopher's bone, flesh and cartilage (BF&C) ointment is also fantastic for these serious injuries. His son David and he were at a convention in the northwest of the United States. A beautiful young lady came up to the booth and said, "How do you like my fingers?" They were nicely groomed, of course, and the Doctor said, "Fine." "Can you tell which finger has been cut off?" she persisted. They couldn't, of course. She said that one of the fingers had been cut off, and she had used the bone, flesh, and cartilage formula, and the knuckle had grown back and the bone and flesh restored. The nail, which had been completely removed, grew back on, and was as pretty as the others.

A similar case: One of Dr. Christopher's neighbors had been in a terrible car accident. Two-thirds of her kneecap had torn off and, although she had other injuries, she worried most about this one. Doctors told her the legs would always be stiff and deformed without the kneecap. She used the BF&C formula and the kneecap grew back. Dr. Christopher was sitting in his former restaurant in the University Mall in Orem, Utah, when a lady came up and said, "Good morning. How do you like my knees?" She pulled her dress up above her knees. He told her they looked fine--a little embarrassed--and asked if they had been damaged. She replied that one had; could he tell which one? She said they were both the same now, because the flesh had been renewed with the BF&C formula. She could bend and squat easily, with perfect functioning of that knee.

One of the most outstanding examples of this formula's use came with a family whose father had really ridiculed Dr. Christopher. He was a businessman, but he liked to fuss with his automobiles. He had taken the motor out of a car, and hoisted it into the air. One of his daughters was playing down on the floor of the garage when something happened to the hoist and it came loose, dropping the car engine on this little girl, mashing her pelvic area and hips. The doctors told her father that the injury was too severe to do anything about. This man had heard about the BF&C formula, and he used it as a fomentation over the entire area where it had been mashed. The particles went jelly-like over a week or two and then started to form. They formed the bones and the pelvic area came back identical to what it was before. As in a jigsaw puzzle, each piece went back into place. This girl went on to live a normal life.

Broken Bones. After a doctor has set the bone, drink three or more cups of bone, flesh, and cartilage and/or comfrey tea or green drink per day. With each cup take two or more capsules of the calcium formula.

Cold Sores. Go on juices, distilled water and red raspberry leaf tea for three days to cleanse the system. C.S.R. formula, green drink, slippery elm gruel, and marshmallow root tea can be given also. Then go on the mucusless diet so the condition will not recur. Use Dr. Christopher's cold sore relief formula (see "Formulas" chapter).

Convulsions. Give tincture of lobelia and/or valerian decoction with a little cayenne. If it comes after a meal, use tincture of lobelia or a finger in the throat to cause vomiting.

Coughs. Make onion syrup by covering several large chopped onions with liquid honey. Low heat under 130 degrees F. for several hours and strain. Hold the syrup in the mouth and let it trickle down. You can also add horehound or wild cherry bark to the honey and onions.

You can massage the chest with antispasmodic tincture, and give a tea made of equal parts wood betony, spearmint, peppermint, and catnip. We usually rub the chest and back with cayenne ointment if a child coughs at night. Almost always, the cough stops till morning.

You can also give the formula for lungs and respiratory tract made by Dr. Christopher; see "Formulas" chapter.

Croup. Give catnip or peppermint tea with a few drops of tincture of lobelia. Give a hot foot bath, followed by a catnip tea enema.

Rub the chest with Professor Cayenne's Deep Heating balm (dilute it with olive oil for young children).

Adjust the person's back.

Earache. Put four to six drops of garlic oil and the same of B tincture into each ear. Stop the ears with cotton.

Place a baked onion on the ear; cut it in half and put a half on each side. Bandage in place and leave on all night.

Use three to six drops of mullein oil in each ear. Rub the oil under and around the ears.

Eruptive Diseases. Give a warm catnip tea enema. Give a hot bath, drinking plenty of catnip, peppermint, red raspberry, yarrow, or elder flowers and peppermint tea. Make sure plenty of liquids are consumed. Hot lemonade (made with fresh lemon and honey), sometimes with minced garlic added, is a wonderful tonic. Give fruit and vegetable juices.

Eye Troubles. If you get a foreign particle in your eye, or if your eyes become red and irritated, you can wash them either with Dr. Christopher's Eyewash, being sure to strain the tea carefully through a fine, clean cotton cloth, or a simple tea of red raspberry leaves. These teas astringe and heal the irritated surface.

Heart Attack. Add a teaspoonful of cayenne to a cup of hot water, and have the patient drink the full cup. Afterward, follow the mucusless diet, hawthorn berry syrup, and bowel formula to cleanse the system and heal the condition. You can drink a daily green drink, adding a tablespoon of wheat germ oil. Keep track of condition by seeing your doctor.

Hiccoughs. Take a good swallow of freshly-squeezed orange juice. Repeat after a few minutes if needed. Dill tea should help. Do a good accupressure treatment on the hands or feet.

Hydrophobia. While sending for a doctor, you can help by doing the following. Press firmly on the vein above the wound to help prevent the poison from ascending. Apply warm water and vinegar to the wound, and when dry, apply a few drops of hydrochloric acid. Then apply a poultice of slippery elm, with a teaspoonful of golden seal, myrrh, and lobelia each added. Change this every couple of hours. You can take an enema to cleanse the colon, followed by a small enema (injection) of lobelia tea. Hold this as long as possible; it will help neutralize the poison in the system. Take golden seal, gentian, myrrh, lobelia and cayenne as a tea--use all or as many of these herbs as you can get. This combination can be helpful in snake bite or insect bite as well. A plantain poultice can help when none of the above is available. But be sure to seek medical help!

Indigestion. This condition can be caused by eating too many acid-forming foods, or by inadequate chewing of food. Remember, "drink your solids," that is, by chewing them fine, and "chew your liquids," swishing them around in the mouth to start digestion.

Peppermint tea can soothe the digestive tract and eliminate gas. Add six to ten drops of lobelia or antispasmodic tincture. Other herbs to soothe the intestinal tract include slippery elm gruel, marshmallow root tea, okra, carrot and spinach juice, and potassium broth.

Dandelion root can gently stimulate liver function which can help digestion. The pancreas formula can sometimes clear up the cause of chronic indigestion.

Insect Stings. Usually the formic acid in an insect sting sets up an irritating and allergic reaction that can be very painful and even cause death in sensitized individuals. Freshly-crushed plantain will reduce the swelling and pain immediately. Plantain ointment is a good second choice. Internally, drink a nervine tea such as scullcap, black cohosh, wood betony, or valerian. Echinacea and tincture of lobelia can be added to the tea.

To prevent insect bites, we have tried nearly every insect repellent on the market. Most of the "organic" ones have not worked too well. The chemicals don't either, except for the army surplus mosquito "dope" we bought in Alaska. It was so strong that it burned the skin.

You can make a decent insect repellent yourself. Combine equal parts of rosemary, basil, wormwood, and rue. Crush well. Add olive oil in proportion of about 1 to 5. Add a spoonful to apple cider vinegar if desired. Set in the sun or over a radiator for a week. Strain well while the moisture is warm. Repeat two more times, the third time let it set a couple weeks or longer if possible. Strain well. This concentrated oil will keep biting bugs away, and it's good for the skin. Apply a dot of it on insect stings, and you'll be surprised at how quickly the swelling and itching will go away.

You can also rub a cut clove of garlic over your skin, eating plenty of raw garlic as well. This does keep the bugs away, but as one seasoned outdoorsman put it, "it keeps everyone else away as well."

Itch. Sometimes itching is caused because toxins are trying to be released from the skin. Use a fomentation made with chickweed tea or plantain, burdock root, Oregon grape root and echinacea, as many of these as you have available, covering it with plastic. Bathe the area with the tea as an alternative, repeating several times a day. Chickweed or plantain ointment can be used on small areas. Drink this in tea as well.

Black walnut tincture can be applied on itching skin. This works especially well if the irritation is due to a fungus or similar invasion. One ounce of powdered golden seal root mixed with nine ounces of pure, food-grade linseed oil (not paint store linseed oil) can be applied externally with good results. White poplar bark tea should be taken internally.

BF&C ointment soothes and heals itching skin, even in the most severe cases.

Lice. Lice should not stay around a body that is clean and perfectly healthy. The mucusless diet and good personal hygiene should keep them away.

When they are present, infuse six parts hyssop, one part walnut leaves or inner bark, one-half part cinnamon powder, one-half part cloves powder, one-half part lobelia, and one-half part ginger. Take a half cup internally three times a day, and make a fomentation over the head and other affected parts with the same formula.

For quick relief, bathe the head or body parts with straight apple cider vinegar, oil of garlic, or black walnut tincture or tea.

Muscle Cramps. Externally, you can apply Professor Cayenne's Ointment. This is very hot, but with a gentle massage, it relaxes tight muscles amazingly fast. Internally, you can mix cramp bark, angelica root, squaw vine, raspberry leaves, chamomile and ginger root and lobelia. Make a tea or wine tincture, and take when cramping. This is also used for menstrual cramps.

Nightmares. Eat light meals only before retiring. Be sure bowels are moving freely. Catnip tea and enema can help a really bad terror. Be selective of daily mental input.

Nosebleed. A teaspoon of cayenne in a cup of hot water will stop most hemorrhages, including nosebleed. To prevent, make sure the body has proper calcium foods. To strengthen the nose membranes, you can inhale a small amount of bayberry bark powder or oak bark powder into the nose. Drink a small amount of the tea of these herbs as well.

Poisons. Call the Poison Control Center to see what therapy should be undertaken. I have found that slippery elm gruel and lobelia together make an excellent poison treatment for non-corrosive poisons. One of our goats ate a poisonous plant and became so sick that she was thought to be as good as dead. By giving her slippery elm and lobelia, her convulsions stopped, and the poison was neutralized. In a few hours she got up, ate and drank. Other common herbs used to combat poisons are arrowroot, balm, bistort, black cohosh, black mustard for narcotic poisoning, borage, coffee, bugbane, chaparral, cornflower, echinacea, elecampane, garlic, gentian, houseleek, juniper berry, marigold, marjoram, mustard, olive oil, parsley, plantain, rue, sassafras, scullcap, sweet basil seeds, white oak, wood betony, wormwood, and yellow flag.

Poison Oak, Poison Ivy. Dr. Christopher used to say that the remedies for these plants grow right near the site of infestation. Burdock leaves and plantain leaves, as well as jewel weed where it grows, can help neutralize the poison. Mullein, houndstongue and lilac leaves will counter the irritation. A poultice of comfrey root, marshmallow root, slippery elm, aloe vera, and witch hazel, as many as you have available and in equal parts, can heal the rash once it starts. Immersion in cold water is very effective. Internally, you can take blood-cleansing and -building herbs, such as chaparral, yellow dock, and echinacea, to help stop the reaction. Internally, lobelia and valerian or catnip or chamomile can stop the pain.

For a **puncture wound.** after cleansing, squeeze until the blood comes out to wash the infection out of the body. Then apply a poultice of freshly crushed plantain leaves. Reapply until wound is healing well. You can use plantain ointment when plantain is not in season. As simple as this is, I have proven it to work. One of my sons stepped on the classic rusty nail, and he has had no tetanus shots. We applied the above procedure, and he had no problem at all.

Shock. Follow the standard first-aid techniques for shock, keeping the patient quiet and warm, and giving liquids if possible. The herbal shock formula, containing one cup of warm water, 1/8 cup honey, one tablespoon apple cider vinegar, and one teaspoon cayenne, works reliably to help bring a person out of shock. The Bach Flower Rescue Remedy works quickly, though subtly, for shock. Massage the feet and hands to help bring circulation to needy areas of the body.

Stiff Neck. Aside from having a chiropractic adjustment, you can massage the neck with the bone, flesh, and cartilage ointment and Professor Cayenne's Deep Heating Balm for immediate relief. Apply a hot fomentation of bone, flesh, and cartilage combination, covering with plastic, each night for healing. You can also drink small amounts of the bone, flesh, and cartilage tea to speed healing.

Sprains. Soak the ankle in a hot foot bath. You can add some fresh, hot comfrey or bone, flesh, and cartilage tea to the bath if you have it. Alternate soaking the sprain in ice cold water. Drink lots of comfrey in tea or green drink. Apply a fomentation of bone, flesh, and cartilage and wrap it securely around the sprain. Use a combination of bone, flesh, and cartilage ointment and Professor Cayenne's Deep

Heating Balm. Take it easy until the pain eases.

Sunburn. Use the burn paste for preference. If it is not available, submerge the sore area in cold water as long as possible. You can also keep cold compresses on the area. Use honey, wheat germ oil or olive oil to saturate the area. Aloe vera gel can promote healing. Some people precede this treatment with a wash of apple cider vinegar.

Toothache. You will likely have to see your dentist, of course, but in the meantime, you can use oil of cloves or oil of peppermint, applied locally, to reduce the pain. You need to supply calcium to the body in an assimilable form right away. You can take Dr. Christopher's calcium formula for this, as well as arrowroot, comfrey, chamomile, chives, dandelion root, flaxseed, horsetail grass, nettle, okra pods, oatstraw, plantain, shepherd's purse.

You can remove the inner membranes from eggshells and soak them in apple cider vinegar after drying and powdering. Let this soak for several days and then add it to distilled water, sweetening with honey. This is an excellent way to feed organic calcium to the system.

Travel. Don't let yourself become dehydrated when you travel. It has been suggested that you drink one cup of water for every hour of flight you undergo. Distilled water is best, although if you are traveling a long distance with a family, this could become impossible! Into your water, put just a drop of ginseng extract. This will help you overcome fatigue. Carry teabags and ask for hot water to make herb tea for yourself. Carry some honey just in case they don't have any. Rose hip tea especially can help you overcome the pollution experienced in airports and cities. Wheat germ oil works in the same way. Carry acidophilus capsules, peppermint teabags, and the lower bowel tonic for digestive disturbances. You can purify your water by soaking wheat grass in it, adding cayenne to it, or having it boiled and making tea out of it. Garlic can help prevent infections and protect you from pollution. A bottle of the Bach Flower Rescue Remedy is a wise adjunct to your travel kit, to ensure that you don't meet something you can't handle.

Be sure to request vegetarian food trays; if you ask for a pure vegetarian food tray, you won't get any dairy products. Take along your cayenne pepper, apple cider vinegar and honey, tamari soy sauce-- whatever you are used to using. These things can help your food digest better and keep the quality of your nutrition up. Bring along some dried fruit, nuts, sprouts and sprouting seeds--whatever you like to snack on. We find that a happy trip, especially with children, revolves around plenty of healthy food available. Only accept pure fruit juices to drink--no soda pop and no alcohol.

Don't forget the ginger root for motion sickness, upset stomach, cramps, etc.

Varicose Veins. Often a person is starved for vital vitamins and minerals, and her system is clogged with mucus from bad food. Dr. Christopher would ask his patients to go on the mucusless diet, and he had wonderful results with the following treatment. He made a strong white oak bark tea, simmering it gently until it reduced by three-fourths. Then he soaked stockings of white cotton in this concentrated tea and asked the patient to wear them, covering them with plastic, all night. He would also paint the legs with the concentrate, if stockings were not available.

Many women had their varicosities reduced miraculously this way.

You can drink a small quantity of this tea as well, if desired.

Worms. Mild cases may respond to eating pumpkin seeds and keeping the bowel clean. Eat one or two ounces of pumpkin seeds daily, and take a tea, steeping an ounce of crushed seeds in a pint of boiling water. Drink a cup or more, up to a pint, six days a week for one to three weeks.

For stubborn worms, use Dr. Christopher's formula for eliminating parasites and worms. Dr. Christopher also recommended this mixture of herbal powders: Equal parts pink root, burdock root, black walnut leaves, male fern, pomegranate root bark, wormwood, and lobelia. Mix the powders and give 1/2 teaspoon of the powder in sorghum molasses or honey. Take each morning and night for three days. On the fourth day, take a cup of three parts senna tea and one part peppermint tea. Repeat after two days' wait. Repeat again.

Eating garlic and placing a peeled button of garlic in the child's rectum six nights a week--or giving garlic enemas--will discourage worms.

MENOPAUSE

What happens when our bodies go into menopause is this: The ovaries begin to cut back on the production of estrogen, which stimulates an increase of a hormone called the follicular stimulating hormone, that which orders the ovaries to start preparing the egg cell. This hormone is trying to get the ovaries to start producing eggs again. The production of this follicular stimulating hormone is normally inhibited because the body produces high enough levels of estrogen. When the level of this hormone increases in the body, it can disturb the hypothalamus gland, which controls normal body temperature, sleep patterns, stamina levels, and control of the autonomic nervous system, which regulates breathing, heartbeat, digestion, blood pressure, and so on. During this gradual adjustment to not producing eggs, these basic functions of the body are disturbed. Few women go through this change without some symptoms.

Only in modern societies has menopause been considered a negative thing. In most other societies, women have welcomed this change as yet another appropriate time in their lives. Many women, wishing to avoid the temporary discomfort of the change, take hormones to continue their periods and delay menopause, although when we stop taking the estrogen, the symptoms simply reappear again; we cannot delay menopause forever. Besides that, estrogen pills carry some pretty frightening side-effects. The labeling on the package insert contains this information, including an increased risk of cancer in the uterus which increases as the time increases that a woman takes the estrogen. Cancer of the breast has also been linked to estrogens. In addition, estrogen does not keep the skin soft or help a woman feel young. It does not help simple nervousness caused by menopause. Other side effects which women have experienced include edema, nausea, dizziness, weight gain, bleeding, vomiting, cramps, nervous tension, and excess cervical secretions.

Various drugs are prescribed for menopausal symptoms, all of them with various unwanted side effects. Rather than list them all, we simply say, avoid all drugs for this natural condition in your body. Natural methods can help you cope with the problem. Some women increase their life's activity and keep themselves busy. They handle their depression and nervousness by working their physical bodies.

Some of them kick the wall or scream when it gets to be too much! Some women rest. Superior nutrition, avoiding undue stress, taking no addictive substances, such as drugs or alcohol, and exercising well can help. Talking over the problems with close friends or relatives can often relieve a bad burden. Some women suggest that our unresolved problems tend to come to the surface when we are experiencing menopause--same as during birth--and it's good to work through these.

Dr. Christopher recalled the case of a lady in Vancouver, B.C. She was climbing the wall with nervous tension due to menopause. Her hot flashes were driving her almost insane. When she would throw off the covers at night, her husband would get cross, as she was keeping him awake at night from her discomfort. She was using estrogen, but she felt it was doing her more harm than good, so she asked Dr. Christopher for help.

He put her on the three-day cleanse and mucusless diet, and she suffered for a time from extreme withdrawal symptoms from taking the commercial hormones. She took the female corrective formula, two or three capsules, three times a day, and the hormone balancing formula, using those three capsules, three times a day. After a short time, she came to Dr. Christopher and said that her whole life had changed. She could sleep all night, without throwing the covers off. She didn't have the nervous screaming jags as she had before, and her husband fell in love with her again. She felt that it was worth the dietary change and the effort to take the herbs to make this difference.

After we go through the menopause, we have experienced another important rite of passage in our womanhood. It signals that our childbearing years are closed, and we enter into a new phase of productivity and experience. Many women feel themselves become more service-oriented, either to their children and grandchildren, or to society, using their talents to enhance others' lives. Some women go to a new career, doing something for the love of it rather than just for need. It's a great time to follow that axiom of working at something you love, and the money will take care of itself. Some women can learn the crafts that they have wished to do all their lives, thus filling their link in the chain of women who have loved to weave, garden, sew, make baskets, dye, etc. In traditional cultures, grandmothers are revered as The Wise Woman, even oracles, of their tribe or society. They can be a very powerful influence.

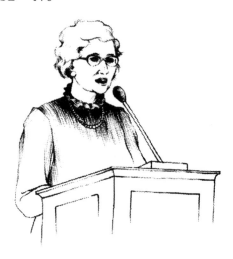

It's also a time to relax in the marriage relationship. Most women say that they do not lose their sexual drive through or after menopause, and it's a time to enjoy the marital relationship without concern about pregnancy.

If we can shed our society's insistent demand that only youth is attractive and worthwhile, we can enjoy this change in our life. I personally think that some of the most beautiful women I've seen are grandmothers.

During menopause, our bodies are doing what they are supposed to be doing, just as they did at puberty, childbearing, and lactation. We can enjoy this, and appreciate the healthy response of our physical mechanism. *Menopause Naturally: Preparing for the Second Half of Life* by Sadja Greenwood, M.D., Volcano Press: San Francisco, 1984, contains a beautifully wholistic approach to the issues of menopause.

THE THREE-DAY CLEANSE, HERBAL CLEANSE, MUCUSLESS DIET AND HERBAL FORMULAS

As you have noticed, the cornerstone of Dr. Christopher's healing methods is the three-day and herbal cleanse combined with the mucusless diet. Most people undertake the three-day cleanse once a month, although it can be repeated more often if the body is highly toxic.

In the morning, drink sixteen ounces of prune juice upon arising. This empties the bowels, and also draws toxic matter from within the entire system.

Throughout the day, we abstain from food and instead take juice of one kind only. Freshly-squeezed juice is much preferred to bottled juice, but pure, unsweetened apple or grape juice can work very well. Whenever you take juice, swish it slowly around in the mouth so it combines well with the saliva and begins digestion. Take a gallon of apple juice--or whatever juice you choose--throughout the day, alternating with pure steam-distilled water. If you become very hungry towards evening, take an apple with the apple juice, a carrot or celery with the carrot juice, etc.

Three times a day take one or two tablespoonsful of olive oil, which helps the liver eliminate toxins.

If your bowels are not moving, either take more prune juice or two or more capsules of the lower bowel tonic three times a day.

Approximately three gallons of toxic lymph will be eliminated from the body, having been replaced by three gallons of alkaline juice.

After the three-day cleanse, start eating food gradually. The first day, eat some fruit for breakfast with one or two tablespoons of finely grated raw almonds. Continue to take your juice through the day, but for lunch you can have a raw salad. For dinner you should have salad again, adding a steamed vegetable.

HERBAL CLEANSE

When dealing with a long-standing health problem, you cannot expect to totally cleanse or cure the body with one or so three-day cleansing routines. Therefore to rid the body of chronic conditions or to prevent their occurrence, an extended herbal cleanse is an excellent path to follow. This should be used in conjunction with the aforementioned mucusless diet.

Upon arising take one or two (more if needed!) of the lower bowel formula. This would then be repeated one hour before lunch, and prior to retiring for the night.

Also, twenty minutes before eating breakfast, take two of the liver-gall bladder formula. Repeat this prior to each meal.

Next on the program take two of the kidney-bladder formula mid-morning and also mid-afternoon. This routine would be followed for six days, resting from the program on the seventh. Resume taking the herbs during the second week, adding two capsules of the blood purifying formula one hour after each meal. Continue using all four formulas at their appointed time each day, six days a week, resting on the seventh day. Continue every week for six weeks, after which you should rest from taking the herbs for a period of one week. Repeat these intervals for six months and then rest from this program for an entire month. At the end of this seven month program, assess your progress and determine if another seven month program would be beneficial.

The one week delay in adding the blood purifying formula is absolutely essential because of the extreme effectiveness of this formula. By using only the lower bowel, liver and gall bladder and kidney and bladder formulas we are opening the eliminative channels of the body, allowing a pathway of elimination for the deeper toxins loosened by the blood cleansing formula.

MUCUSLESS DIET

When you start the mucusless diet, Dr. Christopher suggested some supplements which can speed your healing. Take a teaspoonful of cayenne in cold water three times a day. This is quite a bit to start with, so you should begin with 1/4 teaspoonful and work up to the full amount.

To assist digestion, put one tablespoonful of honey and one of apple cider vinegar in warm water, stirring until mixed. Sip this three times a day. This helps produce hydrochloric acid for digestion.

Use kelp or powdered dulse instead of, or in addition to, sea salt.

This provides many trace minerals and helps the thyroid gland rebuild. You can also take the kelp in tablets. If you cannot stand the taste, try dulse, which is milder, but still wonderfully full of minerals.

Take a tablespoon of molasses three times a day in warm water. You can also take it plain, but the molasses "coffee" is often preferred as a vitamin-B complex pick-me-up.

Take a tablespoonful of a good, fresh wheat germ oil three times a day. This provides vitamin E, which helps the system use oxygen.

See Dr. Christopher's *Regenerative Diet* for charts on sample diets which amply fulfill the RDA recommended for adults and children. Basically, the mucusless diet consists of fruits and vegetables, grains, nuts and seeds. This diet, along with the supplements mentioned above, supply all the nutrients that the body requires. In addition, the high quality of the foods gives new life and health to the system. As we mentioned in the text, some people have been completely healed by the use of the diet alone, although the herbs surely speed recovery.

But what does this diet mean in practical terms? For most of us, it means the elimination of some of our basic foods: milk and milk products, meats, flours--including whole wheat flour but most especially refined flour, sugars, chemicals of all kinds--prepared foods of all kinds.

Instead, we use foods in their wholesome state, fresh, raw or home prepared. Dr. Christopher used an eclectic approach in diet. He didn't recommend all-raw food, because the cooked foods can act as a broom to sweep toxic matter out of the intestines. Cooked food is also familiar and comforting, while a raw diet can be hard to take for many people. He did, however, emphasize using plenty of both raw and cooked foods, not just cooked or just raw.

What do we do with the various categories of foods?

For grains, Dr. Christopher recommended that you soak whole grains in water for sixteen to twenty hours (some say that you should do this in the refrigerator so that the grains will not ferment). Drain off the soak water, and cover with water that has been brought to a boil, along with some sea salt to taste. Low-heat at 135 degrees F. or under (using a food warmer-cooker from a restaurant supply house, a modified crockpot, a stainless steel double boiler, a low temperature in the oven, or a thermos bottle). For the last method, put the soaked grain into the bottle, about 1/3 full. Add the boiling water, turning the thermos a few times so that all the grain is treated. Let this sit all night, and in the morning the grain should be soft and palatable. This only works if you have a small family, however.

You can use wheat, barley, millet, buckwheat, rye, oat groats, and so on. Sprouted grains can also be used.

Some people like to briefly blend the cooked grains in the blender. I especially like this method for children, who do not often chew their food properly.

Serve these grains with a little oil or butter, some honey, some cinnamon, etc. If you are still craving milk on your porridge, soak some almonds overnight. Blend them in the blender with water to cover and one apple, cored but not peeled, and a touch of maple syrup and possibly a bit of pure vanilla. This is so delicious on porridge that you won't miss your milk topping.

You can also slice some fresh fruit, any kind including berries, on your morning cereal. A moderate amount of whole grain bread will not harm you but concentrate on the grains.

During the morning and afternoon, don't hesitate to take a glass of juice (some people like to dilute it, but be sure to swish it around in your mouth), a piece or two of fresh fruit, a few pre-soaked nuts or seeds--whatever you like to snack on. Paavo Airola's research has shown that primitive people in their natural cultures eat a little something every couple of hours or so to keep their energy up. If you are working under real stress, make a "smoothie" by blending soaked almonds, water, honey, pineapple juice, a banana and brewer's yeast together until smooth. This will satisfy your body's needs when demands are high.

We usually prepare a vegetable meal by including something cooked and something raw, something for starch and something for protein. For example, we might steam some zucchini, eat a raw salad, have a baked potato, and have a handful of nuts or a serving of beans. Dr. Christopher recommended using only one cooked vegetable per meal, although you can sometimes prepare more than one. You can vary your vegetables with sauces, herbs, tamari soy sauce, olive oil, a little fresh butter, Vegit, etc. For salad, you can combine almost any vegetables; just be sure not to combine vegetables and fruits, although on occasion you might have a carrot and raisin salad. Dress with olive oil and vinegar, or with homemade mayonnaise.

RECIPES

Mayonnaise

Place in blender:

1	organically-grown egg
2	tablespoons apple cider vinegar, or one T. each vinegar and lemon juice
1	teaspoon salt
1/2	teaspoon ground mustard seed (optional)
1/4	cup unrefined oil (olive and safflower are both good)

Blend on high. Take small cap off blender top and add more oil in a stream until the blender seems to speed up or oil pools on top of mayonnaise. Turn off immediately. If it curdles, take mixture out of blender, clean blender, dry it, start with one egg, and add the mixture to it slowly. It should come out okay. You can also mix this by beating slowly with an egg beater, adding the oil a drop or two at a time, but that method is much more tedious.

You can season the oil-and-vinegar dressing and the mayonnaise almost any way you like. Garlic and basil are good standby seasonings, making an Italian-tasting dressing. But you can add cayenne, almost any herb, more lemon, even natural peanut butter, for different-tasting dressings.

Although you can make salads according to recipes, we usually stick to a miniature salad bar. We prepare raw vegetables as we have them, using leaf lettuce and never iceberg, which has few nutrients but lots of chemicals. We cut or shred what we want, placing the items in nice heaps on a large platter. Each member of the family takes the vegetables that s/he wants. Don't forget to include vegetables that are often served cooked, such as raw, shredded beets--very tasty raw, cauliflower and cabbage, raw peas, etc. Some people eat the starchy vegetables, such as yams and sweet potatoes, raw, but we prefer these cooked. Don't forget a nice little pile of minced garlic, green onions, or chives. Avocados, tomatoes, jicama (a delicious Mexican root vegetable), Jerusalem artichokes, and other unusual vegetables make great, satisfying salads.

For a starch, baked potato is our favorite standby, but baked squash, yams, pumpkins, etc., are also good. You can prepare a grain casserole by mixing soaked, low-heated grains with steamed vegetables. Although this may sound a little plain and mundane, you can come up with some very good combinations, varying seasonings. One of our favorites:

Lentil-Rice Casserole

Soak and low-heat:

2	cups lentils
2	cups brown rice, long or short grain

When the grain is nearly done, add:

2	cups cut carrots, cooked
2	cloves raw garlic
1	large onion, sautéed (optional)
1	bay leaf
1/4	cup blackstrap molasses
2	tablespoons (or more, to taste) apple cider vinegar
2	teaspoons salt

Low-heat for a couple of hours. Makes enough for a large family, or for two hearty meals.

For other grain-casseroles, just add herbs and seasonings with a generous hand. You can lightly toast and grind up some sesame seeds for a lovely topping. Almost any grain and vegetable combination is delicious. *Transfiguration Diet*, by Littlegreen Inc.'s Think Tank, provides detailed recipes and some other information on their application of Dr. Christopher's mucusless diet.

A handful of nuts or seeds, ground up and sprinkled on the vegetables, can provide good protein. You may want to prepare a bean dish, however. Just soak some dried beans for about 24 hours. Then low-heat them until tender, perhaps another 24 hours. You can season them with tomato, garlic, onions, chili, cayenne--almost any seasoning. We love them plain with a little olive oil and tamari sauce; navy beans and garbanzos are delightful this way. You can make soup out of them, or mash them in a pan in which you have heated some oil to make a good dish of refried beans (just be sure to add enough liquid to keep the frijoles creamy). Salt to taste. This simple recipe has a gourmet taste, and it is our family favorite. Most of my children beg me for frijoles refritos!

As you can see, the mucusless diet provides plenty of protein, which is the long-standing lament of those who feel that they can't give up their animal products.

As for nuts and seeds, you can grind them up, mix them with other ingredients, and make a very good confection. For example:

Seed Candy

Sunflower Seeds	Carob Powder
Sesame Seeds	Coconut
Honey	Ground Raisins or other dried fruit (optional)

Grind the seeds in a blender or seed grinder. Add the other ingredients, going light on the honey and adding a touch of water if the mixture needs binding. Roll in more carob powder or sesame seeds or coconut, if desired.

Old-fashioned halvah is nothing but ground sesame seeds and honey, perhaps with a touch of natural vanilla.

Seeds may also be sprouted for use in salads or for eating out of hand. For a long time we enjoyed sunflower seeds out of hand, but when we finally sprouted them, we were amazed at how delicious they are. Soak them overnight, drain them, and in the morning a tiny sprout appears. Sprouted alfalfa seeds are the foundation of many salads, and they are easy to make. Just soak a few tablespoons of alfalfa seeds in water in a wide-mouthed quart jar. Next morning, drain, using a commercial top sold for this purpose, or a nylon stocking, well-cleaned, held on with a jar ring or rubber band. Now rinse the sprouts three times a day or so, letting drain thoroughly each time (that's the secret for sweet sprouts). After four days, they will have grown about three inches long and developed nice green leaves, which you can enhance by leaving the jar for a couple of hours in the sunshine.

Chia seeds make good sprouts, but they are a little gelatinous, which not everyone enjoys. Radish sprouts are spicy and great on salad. Red clover seed sprouts look much like alfalfa but have a slightly different flavor. Mung bean sprouts are sweet and hearty, more starchy than the others, but still great for eating raw. Lentil and garbanzo beans are hefty too. Be sure to cook sprouted soybeans to inactivate the enzyme which makes the bean indigestible.

Some people grow sunflower and buckwheat lettuce by planting the soaked seeds into a small flat of moist soil. This produces tender green leaves which you can clip for salad.

Ann Wigmore suggests a seed cheese which she claims is very digestible. In a blender, blend 1 cup sesame seed, 1 cup sunflower seed, and 2 cups Rejuvelac (see page 143). Put into a muslin bag and allow to drain for 8-12 hours. This is good with vegetables.

Most people can accept the changes required by this diet except for one thing: they want bread. Bread is considered the staff of life (although it's actually wheat that the scripture refers to). Personally, we have had a difficult time giving up bread. You can provide some substitutes, as follows:

Sprout the wheat until the little sprouts appear but no longer. Place the sprouted wheat in a food processor and grind until it forms a bread-like mass. Take this out and place on oiled baking sheet in little loaves. Bake at 150-165° F. for 30 to 60 minutes, or until done to your liking. Slice thin to eat.

Sprout wheat as above, and blend in blender with only a little water until a pancake-batter consistency. Pour onto oiled cookie trays and low-heat as above. Makes a cracker. One family also places the trays under glass frames in the sun; one hot afternoon should give you good crackers.

Both of the above recipes can be sweetened with honey, lightly salted, or flavored with herbs or ground raisins.

If you are still hankering after regular bread, you can make an improvement on your regular whole wheat loaves by sprouting the wheat as above, perhaps a quart of sprouts, and blending with a very little water in the blender. Use this as the base of your whole wheat bread, adding it to activated yeast, a little honey (though not very much, because the sprouting process makes the wheat very sweet), some sea salt, and adding only as much whole wheat flour as you need to knead the loaf. One baker also adds a cup or two of gluten flour, which is very concentrated, but does really improve the texture. Knead, rise and bake as usual. Although this is not a live food, the acidity of much of the grain is changed to alkaline and the bread is better for us. However, the texture is very heavy and somewhat sticky, not at all like the light fluffy bread we're used to. Still, it's a trade-off, because whole wheat bread as we normally consume it is very mucus-forming, a dead food.

One nutritionist suggests that if you must have bread, you should bake pita bread and then stuff it with good salad vegetables, including avocado if you can. Add plenty of sprouts, and this perhaps will balance the acidifying effect of the bread.

Pita

2 cups warm water
2 tablespoons honey
1 tablespoon dried yeast
Activate yeast

Add:
1 teaspoon sea salt
1 teaspoon kelp (optional)

Mix in:
5-6 cups of freshly-ground whole wheat flour, as needed to make a dough that you can knead

Flour a clean surface, and knead until springy. Let rest 15 minutes.
Break off golf-ball sized pieces of dough, and roll out about 1/4 inch thick into tortilla-shaped circles. Place on ungreased cookie sheet that has been sprinkled with cornmeal. Let rise about 30 minutes, during which you preheat your oven to 450° F.
Place sheets on bottom shelf of oven, and bake the pita breads for 5-8 minutes, just until they puff and solidify a bit. Remove and cool separately. If you don't have a lot of cookie sheets, let the breads rise on a cornmeal-sprinkled surface, and gently, gently place them on the cookie sheets as they become available. Makes 2 dozen pita breads. Cut

in half across the circle to form two pockets and stuff as desired. Homemade mayonnaise is a good dressing.

Another frustration in adapting to this diet is the absence of milk. But to heal quickly, and especially for serious disease, it's best to eliminate milks entirely. However, you can make palatable nut and seed milks that behave quite a bit like milk. Just blend (soaked) almonds in water, in proportions of about one to four. Blend until smooth and strain if desired, although we enjoy the pulp as well. Sesame and coconut also make good milks. Sunflower seed milk is strongly flavored but still pleasant.

You can make soy milk, which many people use as a plentiful milk substitute. The best-tasting recipe we have seen is as follows:

Soy milk

Sort through 1 quart dry soybeans and discard bad ones. Soak overnight in three cups of water. Drain well.

Put on a large pot of water to boil. In a blender which you have preheated by blending 2 cups of boiling water for 1 minute, put in 1 cup of beans to the 2 cups of boiling water. Grind for 2 or 3 minutes. Strain in a muslin bag to remove the pulp, and squeeze well to get out as much of the milk as you can.

Heat the milk at least 30 minutes in a double boiler. Stir occasionally.

Add 2 tablespoons oil, and a little honey, if desired. Refrigerate and use as dairy milk.

The flavor of this milk is mild and pleasant. You should be careful not to crack a plastic or glass blender container with the boiling water.

Some people enjoy sprouted-wheat milk, which is made by blending sprouted wheat with water until creamy. It's a little strong-tasting but very satisfying.

Sometimes a little apple or grape juice over grains or other fruits can be delicious and satisfying.

The only safe sweeteners are honey, blackstrap molasses, sorghum, maple syrup, or fruit sugars (that is, ground-up dried fruits, such as date). Any processed sugars should be avoided. They are often the main cause of many health problems.

In the evening or between meals, fruits can be very satisfying. A large bowl of chopped fruits of various kinds, sprinkled with wheat germ, ground nuts or seeds, or a bit of honey, is a delectable treat. You can use avocado with fruits or vegetables, making a rich and satisfying meal.

Dr. Christopher recommended using a potassium broth with vegetable meals. This is most easily made by purchasing Dr. Jensen's or Dr. Bonner's broth. However, we like to make our own. Just simmer potatoes, celery, carrots, onions, garlic, herbs and whatever other vegetables you like in water until tender. When it's done, add tamari soy sauce to taste. You can blend this in the blender if you like. This simple recipe is very delicious and satisfying.

You can make delicious soups by blending fresh, raw vegetables (only good-quality, good-tasting ones that you'd normally eat raw) with hot water or nut or soymilk. Just clean and cut up the vegetables (corn, peas, tomatoes, celery, carrot, etc.) and place them in the blender with seasonings and hot water. Blend until smooth and serve immediately. You might need to warm it up a little on the stove. A little well-sautéed onion makes the soup taste cooked. Our favorite variation of the raw soup is eaten cold:

Summer Soup or Gazpacho

In the blender container place:

Several cut-up, ripe tomatoes
1   clove garlic, peeled
1   stick celery, cut-up
1   green pepper, cleaned and cup up
2   teaspoons basil or 2 tablespoons fresh basil
1   teaspoon sea salt
1/2   teaspoon paprika

Blend until smooth, strain through a colander, and serve cold.

Some people like to purchase or make a nutmeat preparation to stand-in for meats.

Nut Loaf

1	part cashews, coarsely ground
1	part almonds, coarsely ground
1	part celery, finely chopped
1	part carrots, finely chopped
1/4	part minced parsley
1	part tomato, blended in blender or finely chopped
1	avocado, mashed
	salt, pepper, herbs, Vegesal, etc., to taste

Mix all together and press into loaf pan. Refrigerate until firm.

You can buy vegetarian meat substitutes, but check the labels for additives. Once we bought some meatless hot dogs, and they contained nitrates and nitrites the same as the meat variety!

You can also make bean loaves by combining beans, crumbs, vegetables, and seasonings, baking for a half hour if desired.

We tend to go more simple than this, however, simply using the foods as they are without making too many combinations.

As for sauces, you can make a lovely off-white sauce by using olive oil or butter, whole-wheat flour, and almond milk. Flavor this as desired. Just alter your regular sauce recipes using the foods recommended in this diet.

Make vegetarian burgers with tofu by mixing; chopped onion, 1 egg, mashed tofu or pinto beans, shoyu or tamarri sauce and oatmeal to bind. Cook on oiled griddle. They're very good substitutes for hamburgers.

Desserts are hard to give up, but you can alter some of your favorite recipes so they are mucusless and delicious. In Dr. Christopher's *Regenerative Diet*, a pudding is suggested:

Strawberry Barley Pudding

Strawberry Barley Pudding is an elegant spoon-up finish for any luncheon or dinner. And leftovers are quite a temptation to any refrigerator raider. Try this appealing and delicious delight.

2   cups strawberries
2   cups low-heated barley
1/2   cup honey
1/2   teaspoon almond extract

Combine above ingredients in blender, purée and set aside.

2   cups strawberries
1/2   cup honey
2   tablespoons arrowroot
1/2   teaspoon almond extract

Combine these ingredients in the top of a double boiler. Heat to 130° F. and maintain heat for 30 minutes. Remove from heat and add barley mixture from blender.

Place in refrigerator and chill thoroughly. Just before serving top with coconut chips and garnish with fresh strawberry halves.

This method of making pudding can be adapted to other fruits and grains, varying flavors as desired.

You can make a nice fruit cobbler by lightly steaming fresh fruit, sweetening as desired, and topping with ground, low-heated grains, lightly-toasted and ground seeds or nuts, lightly-toasted wheat germ, etc. Top with nut cream, which is just nut milk made with a little less water, sweetened with honey or maple syrup.

These are just a few recipes we enjoy. More can be found in *The Mild Food Cookbook* by Michael Tracy, which offers simple recipes that make the mucusless diet delicious.

You may question the cost of such a diet. Actually, if you eliminate the high-prices processed foods from your grocery list, you free up quite a bit of money that can be used to bring home much delicious, fresh produce. Even if it does cost more than you are used to paying, you will be eliminating visits to the doctor's office, supplements at the health food store, and time lost from work. I consider our grocery budget money invested in health. Once we bought several bags of fruit when we lived in Toronto, Canada. The check-out attendant asked us if we worked for a restaurant!

During the winter, you can usually obtain good vegetables and fruits in most parts of the country, although in some places, such as Alaska, the price can get pretty high. I always wonder what we would do if shipping were somehow stopped, as in an economic disaster. I would hope that we could contrive some sort of storage facility, such as an underground pit. I have seen people store carrots, celery, squash, apples, pears, etc., in root cellars all the way through until the next harvest, and in good condition, too. Dr. Christopher always recommended that people grow their own food, experimenting with varieties that are not necessarily "supposed" to grow in their locales. He recalled that his father had the first bearing almond tree in Salt Lake City, Utah. Everyone else thought they couldn't grow there.

A mainstay of the winter mucusless diet must be sprouts. If you can accustom your family to eating sprouts, they can form an important part of your salads, and soups too. Ann Wigmore suggests a soup made of your favorite sprouts, plus buckwheat lettuce and sunflower greens. Blend this with seasonings and water in your blender, and it makes a high-powered, nutritious soup.

As you begin the mucusless diet, you will feel yourself getting more and more energy and needing less and less food. Sometimes you may be tempted to go off the diet, but you might try this trick offered by a nutritionist. When you feel reasonable tempted by ice cream, chocolate, or some other forbidden food, take just one bite and chew it slowly. Then ask yourself, do you really want more of this? If you feel strongly that you do, take just one more bite and repeat. Often the body's mechanism will deny the need for the food once it gets the vibrations of what's going in. In any case, don't allow yourself to shovel in bad food. Go for a walk if you have to! Take a couple of glasses of cold water. You can eventually overcome bad food cravings.

During the process of cleansing and rebuilding your body, you can expect what is called a cleansing crisis. Your symptoms may all flare up; you may feel bad all over; you may feel like you have the flu. Just keep going, the cleansing crisis will pass, and you'll feel better than ever. Dr. Christopher used to have recurrent flare-ups of his rheumatism and arthritis; for a week or two every seven years he would have to go back to his wheelchair. He accepted these crises, as hard as they were to live with, and continued on with the business of cleansing and building his body.

Look upon your new adventure in diet as fun, interesting, and freedom-giving. You will gain your health from it, and also learn to control the sources and preparation of your food. Take it for granted that the food tastes good, that it's good for you, and that it's making you better. Soon you'll be delighted at how good it tastes and how much you enjoy it; it will become a way of life.

FORMULAS

We have referred to many of Dr. Christopher's herbal formulas. Unlike many practitioners, Dr. Christopher shared the contents of his formulas freely with others. We are happy to share the ingredients with you.

Provided herein are 61 basic cleansing and rebuilding herbal formulas. These combinations have been formulated with the average individual in mind and meet nearly all general problem requirements. Consult a competent health practitioner for any uncommon health problems not found within the scope of these formulas. These formulas are not intended to be used as a replacement for competent medical attention but within a full health program.

Listed below each formula are the names used by various vendors who supply Dr. Christopher's products. His formulas are the most widely distributed in the United States. If you cannot find a particular formula in you local health food store, you can call: The Herb Shop at 1-800-453-1406 or P. O. Box 777 Springville, UT 84663.

1. Lower bowel formula.
Barberry bark (*Berberis vulgaris*)
Cascara sagrada bark (*Rhamnus purshiana*)
Cayenne (*Capsicum fastigiatum, Capsicum minimum*)
Ginger (*Zingiber officinale*)
Lobelia herb and/or seeds (*Lobelia inflata*)
Red raspberry leaves (*Rubus idaeus*)

Turkey rhubarb root (*Rheum palmatum*)
Fennel (*Foeniculum vulgaris*)
Golden seal root (*Hydrastis canadensis*)

Take according to how many you need. As there are no two people alike in age, size, or physical construction (and the bowel itself will differ in persons as much as the finger prints), most cases will START with two number 0 capsules or 30 drops of the glycerine based extract three times a day, and then regulate the dosage from there. If the stool seems too loose then cut down, but if it is difficult to get a bowel movement and the stool is hard and takes a long time, then increase the amount until the movements become soft and well-formed (and here, in very difficult cases, you could take even up to 40 of these capsules a day, for these herbs are only FOOD and can do no damage to you).

After the hard material has broken loose and is eliminated (these are hard incrustations of fecal matter that have been "stored" in the bowel for many years that are breaking loose and soaking up intestinal liquids), you can gradually decrease but do not taper off the lower bowel formula dosage so much at this point that you lose this advantageous momentum and continuity of elimination. In most cases, the improper diet has caused the peristaltic muscles of most people to quit working, and it will take six to nine months with the aid of the lower bowel formula for the average individual to clean out the fecal matter and to rebuild the bowel structure sufficiently to have the peristaltic muscles work entirely on their own.

Most people have pounds of old dried fecal matter that is stored in the colon which is toxifying the system and keeping the food from being assimilated--because of this putrified condition, most people engorge themselves with many times more food than the actual body requirements. In the process they wear out their bodies in trying to get sufficient nutrition and are still always hungry and eating; whereas, after the bowel is cleaned, the food is readily assimilated and a person can sustain himself on about one-third the quantity of his current food consumption at some four or five times more power, vitality and life. Herein, the clean body is able to normally assimilate the simple food values through the cell structures in the colon instead of it being trapped in a maze of waste and inhibited by the hard fecal casing on the intestinal wall, which causes the large part of nutrition to be pushed on and eliminated before it can do any good. When the body is completely clean, these aids will no longer be necessary--then your food will be your medicine and your medicine will be your food. After following this program properly and the bowel is cleansed, this formula should only be used when needed. Sources: Herbal L.B., FEN LB, Naturalax 2.

2. Blood Purifying formula. The blood stream is life itself and it is our job to keep it clean and pure so that we can have a good circulatory system for delivering food to the body properly, and, in addition, to carry off the waste materials.

After years of using this blood purifying formula, we discovered it to be the same type formula as used by Hoxey.

This herbal blood rebuilder is made up of herbs that are cleansers, herbs that give astringency, others aid in removing cholesterol, kill infection, and build elasticity in the veins and strengthen the vein and artery walls. It consists of red clover blossoms, chaparral, licorice root, poke root, peach bark, Oregon grape root, stillingia, cascara sagrada, sarsaparilla, prickly ash bark, burdock root and buckthorn bark.

Use a cup of this tea or two capsules No. 0 or 5 to 15 drops of the glycerine based extract three time a day, six days a week, week after week, until the blood stream is flowing as it should to bring health and give one more pep and energy.

This blood purifier in teamwork with the bowel cleansing and rebuilding formula, the liver-gall bladder formula and the kidney formula, makes a wonderful combination. These four, with a good mucusless diet, can renew the body and add years to a healthy life. (See section on "Herbal Cleanse," page 171). Sources: Red Clover Combination, R.C.C.

3. Liver and Gall Bladder formula. To speed up the blood purifying process, it is good to have a clean liver and gall bladder area. When the liver does not function properly, the bile does not excrete freely into the intestinal tract, and so it passes off into the blood stream and throughout the rest of the system, causing a toxic condition called cholemia, causing indigestion, sluggishness, fatigue, constipation, upset stomach, chills, vomiting and fever. Why wait until it gets to this condition? A combination of barberry (or Oregon grape root) and each of the following herbs--wild yam, cramp bark, fennel seed, ginger, catnip and peppermint will help relieve this condition.

Suggested dose: 1cup of the tea or one or two capsules or 15 to 30 drops of the glycerine based extract, 15 or 20 minutes before a meal. Sources: Barberry LG, Hepatean, LG

4. Kidney and Bladder formula. Approximately 80% of the body is liquid, and much of this fluid must be pumped, filtered, etc., through the urinary system of the individual. We generally do not take the best care of this delicate tract. Through it circulates irritating and clogging-type materials, i.e., tea, coffee, soft drinks, hard water, alcohol, etc.

Over the years we have used a formula of herbs with people who have been afraid to be out in public because of lack of control over the urinary tract and unknowingly voiding urine. After using this formula, many people have found relief from this condition and are living normal lives again.

This formula consists of juniper berries, parsley, uva ursi, marshmallow root, lobelia, ginger, and golden seal. Suggested use is a cup of tea morning and evening, or two capsules or 30 to 60 drops of the glycerine based extract morning and evening taken with a cup of parsley tea. Sources: Juni-Pars, Renatean, KB.

5. Bed Wetting formula. For more severe cases of incontinence, neurosis (bed wetting, etc.), a formula we have used a long time is as follows: parsley root, juniper berries, marshmallow root, white pond lily, gravel root, uva ursi, lobelia, ginger root and black cohosh root.

This formula is a specific for controlling or overcoming bed wetting and to strengthen the entire urethral canal, kidneys, bladder, etc.

Recommended dosage: Two No. 0 capsules three times a day with a cup of parsley tea. Upon retiring at night fasten about a six or eight inch ball of yarn or string or cloth onto night clothes in the middle of the back. This is for the purpose of preventing the individual from lying on the back, as this is generally the time the valves release to void urine. Sources: DRI.

6. Heart formula. The heart is our life pump, and when it is not properly fed (with wholesome foods) it suffers malfunction (weakness and heart attacks) causing the heart failure condition that is one of the worlds greatest killers. The mucusless diet used over a period of time can rebuild a heart to a good strong condition, but if the heart, its valves, and other working parts are in a weakened condition and need quick help we use a great heart food or tonic to assist it back to health. This food is the hawthorn berry (*Crataegus oxycantha*, Linn.). We refer back to *Potters Cyclopaedia of Botanical Drugs and Preparations*, one of the old herbals out of England (published by Potter and Clarke, Ltd., 60 Artillery Lane, London), which lists hawthorn as a "cardiac" tonic. This herb is claimed to be a curative remedy for organic and functional heart disorders such as dyspnoea, rapid and feeble heart action, hypertrophy, (valvular insufficiency), and heart oppression.

Hawthorn berry syrup is made with hawthorn berry juice concentrate using grape brandy and glycerine as aids and preservatives. Recommended dosage is one half teaspoon three times a day.

In an emergency heart attack, a teaspoon of cayenne in a cup of hot water taken quickly has saved many peoples lives. To save time, the extract should be kept on hand. Sources: Hawthorn Berry Syrup.

7. Pancreas formula and other affiliated glands that through malfunction cause high or low blood sugar (namely diabetes or hypoglycemia). This combination has assisted many that have had hypoglycemia. Use two or three capsules or 15 to 30 drops of the glycerine based extract three times a day, six days a week. (All herbal aids give faster results in six days a week instead of seven, using the same days of each week.) Many have had a glucose tolerance test with a clean bill of health on the pancreas area. Many reports have come in about heavy insulin users who continue using the insulin but by watching litmus paper or other types of diabetic checking have gradually tapered down on the insulin; and many within a year, have found complete relief using two to three or more capsules, or 30 to 60 drops of the glycerine based extract of the pancreas formula three times a day, six days a week. Of course, the closer a person stays on the mucusless diet and eliminates from the diet the unnatural sugars, soft drinks, candies, pastries, bread, etc., the quicker the results. The herbal formula is golden seal, uva ursi, cayenne, cedar berries, licorice root and mullein. Sources: Panc Tea, Pancreatean, PC.

8. Calcium formula. A wonderful natural calcium capsule, tea or glycerine based extract made up of six parts horsetail grass, three parts oat straw, four parts comfrey root and lobelia. As explained in the book Biological Transmutations, the silica in horsetail grass converts to calcium, and the other herbs work in close conjunction with this master calcium herb. We need calcium for nerve sheath, vein and artery walls, bone, teeth, etc. This combination is all pure herbs. It is also used for cramps, charlie horses, and for all calcium needs in the body.

Children with crowded, crooked teeth who later must have the wisdom teeth pulled because their jaw is too narrow are lacking calcium in the body. The pregnant woman should increase her natural calcium intake now for two people, so as to build for the child a good wide jaw and tooth material. Sugars, pastries, soft and alcoholic beverages, breads, candies, etc., leach the calcium out of the body, causing varicose veins, cramps, charlie horses, loss of teeth, nervous upsets, etc. Sources: Calc Tea, Calctean, Kid-E-Calc, CA-T.

9. Allergies, Sinus, and Hayfever formula. This is an aid for clearing up these malfunctions, a natural and herbal help working as a decongestant and natural antihistamine to dry up the sinuses and expel from the head and bronchial-pulmonary tubes and passages the offending stoppage and mucus. This formula consists of the following herbs: Brigham tea, marshmallow root, golden seal root, chaparral, burdock root, parsley root, lobelia and cayenne. Take two capsules or 20 to 40 drops of the glycerine based extract three times a day or as often as needed.

To speed up this cleansing procedure, use the following combination in addition to the above: Blend fresh, chopped-up horseradish roots mixed with apple cider vinegar into a thick pulp and chew thoroughly before swallowing. Take 1/3 teaspoon three times in a day. Increase this amount 1/3 teaspoon each three days, up to one teaspoon three times a day. (For a sinus preparation that contains horseradish, see formula #58 on page 203). Sources: SHA Tea, Sinutean, HAS.

10. Blood Pressure formula. This group of herbs feeds cayenne (a stimulant) and ginger (stimulant) into the circulatory system where the cayenne works from the bloodstream to the heart and arteries and out into the veins. The other herbs in the formula assist these two herbs and work together to equalize the blood pressure (whether high or low) bringing it to a good systolic over the diastolic reading. Blood flow is life itself. This formula is given to assist blood purifying teas to work more efficiently and to also aid the clearing up of allergies, etc. The blood circulatory combination consists of ginger, cayenne, golden seal, ginseng, parsley and garlic. (Available in capsules and glycerine based extract). Sources: BPE, Circutean, B/P.

11. Anti-Obese Herbal Food formula. Combine this anti-obese aid with the mucusless diet and you have a winner. This is not a crash program for fast loss of weight, but graduated and accurate loss without robbing the body of the needed nutrients like so many fad diets do. This acts as a blood purifier, aids kidneys in relieving excess fluids, feeds the body for relief from nervous tension generally caused by diets, appeases the appetite, feeds the thyroid and other malfunctioning glands and thus gains a healthier state for holding weight control. Take two or three capsules morning and night with a cup of chickweed tea. The formula is chickweed, burdock, licorice, saffron, mandrake, fennel, parsley root, kelp, echinacea, black walnut, hawthorn berries and papaya. Sources: CSK Plus, SLM.

12. Malfunctioning Glands formula. Through the accumulation of toxic waste in the body from improper diet, poor blood stream and sluggish circulation, the glands become congested and infected and swell up to cause much pain and misery. (There are glands that swell on the neck, breast, groin, under arm, etc.) Make a tea of three parts mullein and one part lobelia herb and use as a fomentation over swollen or malfunctioning glands. Leave on all night (covering fomentation with plastic), six nights a week until relief is obtained. Use a fresh fomentation as warm as possible each night.

This can be used as an aid to relieve mastitis, thyroid malfunction, etc. In addition to the external fomentation, also drink a cup of this tea two or three times a day or take two of the capsules with a cup of steam-distilled water. Source: Mullein & Lobelia.

13. Nerve Herbal Food formula. Here is a formula we have used with great success for well over thirty years and is used for relieving nervous tension and insomnia. It is mildly stimulating and yet lessens the irritability and excitement of the nervous system, and also lessens or reduces pain. This formula contains herbs that feed and revitalize the motor nerve at the base of the skull (medulla area and upper cervicals), and also herbs that help rebuild or feed the spinal cord. This group of herbs will also rebuild the frayed nerve sheath, the nerve itself, and its capillaries.

The following herbs in this combination are food for your valuable--and in many cases, shattered nerves: black cohosh, capsicum, hops flowers, lobelia, skullcap, valerian, wood betony and mistletoe. The suggested amount for an adults use would be one to three cups of the tea, or two or three capsules, or 15 to 30 drops of the glycerine based extract, three times a day, taken with a cup of celery juice or steam-distilled water. Sources: Relax-Eze, Nervean, Ex-Stress.

14. Hearing Loss and Earache formula. When this procedure is used as explained here, it can be an aid in assisting an improvement of poor equilibrium, failure of hearing, aiding the motor nerve, etc. With an eye dropper put into each ear at night four to six drops of olive oil based garlic extract and four to six drops of the herb tincture listed below, plugging ears overnight with cotton, six days a week, four to six months, or as needed. On the seventh day, flush ears with a small ear syringe using warm apple cider vinegar and distilled water half and half. The herb tincture is made of blue cohosh, black cohosh, blue vervain, skullcap and lobelia. Source: B&B and Oil of Garlic.

15. Lungs and Respiratory Tract formula. This combination of herbs is an aid to relieve irritation in the respiratory tract, lungs and bronchials. This is an aid in emphysema as well as other bronchial and lung congestions such as bronchitis, asthma, tuberculosis, etc. This formula is extremely valuable in strengthening and healing the entire respiratory tract. It promotes the discharge of mucus secretions from the bronchio-pulmonary passages. Suggested amount for an adult is a cup of tea two or three times a day, or two or three capsules or 10 to 20 drops of the glycerine based extract two or three times a day with a cup of comfrey tea. For additional help in the program, it is good to add three to six drops of tincture of lobelia to each cup of tea.

This formula consists of comfrey root, mullein, chickweed, marshmallow root and lobelia. Sources: Resp-Free, Respratean, Breathe-Aid.

16. Colds and Infections formula. This combination of garlic, parsley, watercress, rosemary and rosehips acts as an aid to assist in relieving colds, etc., or wherever garlic is needed to help stop infection! The adult amount can vary from one to six or more cups in a day or two or more capsules six or more times per day taken with a cup of steam-distilled water. Sources: Garlic, Rosehips & Parsley; Winter Formula C&F.

17. Intestinal Parasites formula. This combination of wormwood, American wormseed, tame sage, fennel, malefern and papaya acts as a vermifuge (herbal agent that will cause expulsion of worms and parasites from the body) and/or vermicide (herbal agent that destroys worms and parasites in the body). Recommended dosage is to take one teaspoon each morning and night for three days. On the fourth day drink one cup of senna and peppermint tea, using teaspoon of each in a cup of hot, distilled water. Rest two days and repeat two more times. Source: VF Syrup.

18. Tooth Powder formula. This herbal food combination consists of oak bark, comfrey root, horsetail grass, lobelia, cloves, and peppermint. This formula is used to help strengthen the gums (bleeding and pyorrhea-type infections of the gums), and assist in tightening loose teeth. This type of tooth powder will brighten tooth luster and make for a healthier mouth.

For severe cases place this powder combination between the lips and gums (upper and lower) around entire tooth area and leave on all night, six nights a week (as well as brushing regularly) until improvement is evident. Then continue on with regular brushing with this herbal food combination. Source: Herbal Tooth Powder

19. Composition Powder formula. This herbal food combination consists of bayberry bark, cloves, ginger root, cayenne and white pine bark. As quoted by Dr. Nowell, our instructor at the Dominion Herbal College, Ltd. of Vancouver, British Columbia in our textbook:
"We have made and used composition powder for over forty years. When we state we regularly mixed it in batches of sixty pounds the student will readily see that we have had at least some experience with it. As a remedy in colds,

beginning of fevers, flu, hoarseness, sluggish circulation, colic, cramps, etc. We believe it has done more good than any other single preparation ever known to man.

If this compound were kept in every home, and used as the occasion arose, there would be far less sickness. Give it freely in your practice and your patient will bless you. Look over the ingredients, and consider how it will clear canker, ease cramps and pains in the stomach and bowels, raise the heat of the body equalizing the circulation, and removing congestions. It is safe. It is effective. We have on numberless occasions given a cup of composition tea every hour as warm as the patient could drink it, until the patient has perspired freely, and after four or five doses have seen our patients in a free perspiration, thereby removing colds and febrile trouble."

Source: Herbal Composition

20. Eyewash formula. This formula is excellent for brightening and healing the eyes, and it is known to remove the cataracts and heavy film from the eyes: bayberry bark, eyebright herb, golden seal root, red raspberry leaves, and cayenne. Using the powder or the extract, make into tea form and put into an eye cup made of glass. There will be a burning sensation when using the eyewash at first. This is due to the stimulating effect of the cayenne pepper and will do nothing but good to the eyes. Tip head back and apply the eye cup to eye. Exercise eye while doing this as though you were swimming under water. Do this three to six times a day and take two capsules or a cup of the tea, morning and evening. Source: Herbal Eyebright Powder and Extract.

21. Female Corrective formula. This is an amazing combination of herbs to aid in rebuilding a malfunctioning reproductive system (uterus, ovaries, fallopian tubes, etc.). Over the years herbalists and patients have seen painful menstruations, heavy flowing, cramps, irregularity, etc., change to a painless menstrual period, good menstrual timing, and a new outlook on life by using these aids to readjust the malfunctioning areas. This herbal aid for female reproductive organs consists of golden seal root, blessed thistle, cayenne, cramp bark, false unicorn root, ginger, red raspberry leaves, squaw vine and uva ursi.

Recommended dosage is one cup of tea or two capsules or 30 to 60 drops of glycerine based extract three times a day or more if desired, six days a week for as long as required to get the desired results. We have seen many severe cases who have had many years of suffering cleared up in ninety to 120 days. Some get relief sooner, some take longer--no two cases are alike. This is a food to rebuild the malfunctioning organs. Sources: Nu Fem, FEM.

22. Prostate Area formula. In case of malfunction we suggest this combination to assist the male: cayenne, ginger, golden seal root, gravel root or queen of the meadow root, juniper berries, marshmallow root, parsley root or herb, uva ursi leaves and ginseng. This will dissolve the stones that are in the kidneys, as well as clean out other sedimentation and infection in the prostate. Mix the powders and place in No. 0 capsules and take two or more morning and night, with parsley tea when possible. Sources: Prospallate, PR.

23. Hormone Balancing formula. These are natural herbal foods that are needed by both men and women at all ages. Being natural herbs, the human body can accept, assimilate and use these needed materials to produce estrogens and other hormones naturally. This formula will assist in rebuilding the weak malfunctioning areas and help keep the organs healthy so they can supply the proper amounts of hormones and estrogens themselves. The critical times when this formula is necessary, are when entering puberty, during pregnancy, during the weeks and sometimes months following the birth of a child, and during menopause. Herbs are a natural food, so they do not have "side effects" and "after effects" as are so evident in man-made synthetic drugs. Herbs used in this formula are black cohosh, sarsaparilla, ginseng, licorice, false unicorn, holy thistle and squaw vine.
    Whenever malfunction shows in the female reproductive areas, it is good to use formulas No. 21 and No. 23 together. For male reproductive problems use formulas No. 22 and No. 23 together. Sources: Changease, Fematean, Change-O-Life.

24. Herbal Bolus formula. Here is another excellent aid for both men and women who have problems in the reproductive areas. Boluses are made with healing herbs that feed malnourished organs and draw out the toxins and poisons making the malfunctioning area clean and healthy, so that scavengers like cysts, tumors, and cancerous conditions will not have waste material to survive on or live in.

Herbalists who use this formula have found that these scavengers will release and be eliminated. The bolus spreads its herbal influence widely from the vagina or bowel through the entire urinary and genital organs. The formula consists of powered: squaw vine herb, slippery elm bark, yellow dock root, comfrey root, marshmallow root, chickweed herb, golden seal root and mullein leaves.

Coconut butter should be melted down so that it will mix well with the herb powder. Mix a small quantity of this powder, and wet to pie dough consistency with coconut butter (which can be purchased from the drug store, health food store, or herb shop). Next, roll this mass between hands until you have a pencil-like bolus approximately the size of the middle finger in about inch-long pieces. Harden in a refrigerator. These are to be inserted into the vagina or rectum much the same as suppositories would be. It may be necessary to wear a sanitary napkin.

Insert upon retiring and leave in all night, six nights a week. The coconut butter melts at body temperature, leaving only the herbs, and these are easy to douche out. The following morning use the routine in formula #25. Sources: V.B., Herbal Bolus.

25. Prolapse Organ formula. To build and relieve prolapsed uterus, bowel, or other organs or for hemorrhoid problems, make a concentrated tea (simmer down to half its amount) of this formula containing: oak bark, mullein herb, yellow dock root, walnut bark or leaves, comfrey root, lobelia and marshmallow root. Inject with a syringe (while head down on a slant board) into vagina or rectum, to cup or more. Leave in as long as possible before voiding. When the tea is injected into the abdominal area and while on the slant board, knead and massage the pelvic and abdominal area to exercise muscles, so the herbal tea (food) will be assimilated into the organs. It is helpful to drink one fourth cup of tea concentrate in three fourths cup of distilled water three times a day or take 2 capsules three times a day. Sources: Yellow Dock Combination.

26. Anti-Miscarriage formula. The anti-miscarriage formula consists of these two herbs: false unicorn and lobelia. Unless otherwise specified, teas are always made with one teaspoon of herbs to a cup of distilled water if obtainable. If hemorrhaging starts during pregnancy, stay in bed, use a bed pan when needed, and drink a cup of the tea each hour until bleeding stops, continue drinking a cup each waking hour for one day, while in bed as much as possible, and then a cup three times a day for three weeks. If bleeding continues instead of decreasing, see a doctor. Source: False Unicorn & Lobelia.

27. Prenatal formula. Using this tea (or two or three capsules) morning and evening is an aid in giving elasticity to the pelvic and vaginal area and strengthening the reproductive organs for easier delivery. The formula should be used only in the last six weeks before time of birth as follows: 1 capsule per day of the first week, 2 capsules per day the second week and 2 capsules three times a day from the third week on. 6 capsules a day is the maximum dosage suggested. The herbs used in this combination are: squaw vine, holy thistle, black cohosh, pennyroyal, false unicorn, raspberry leaves and lobelia. Source: Pre-Natal Tea, PN-6.

28. Bone, Flesh, and Cartilage formula or the comfrey combination. This is an aid for malfunction in bone, flesh, cartilage, and is excellent for varicose veins, sprains, curvature of the spine, tremors, skin eruptions, pulled muscles, blood clots, calcium spurs, etc. This combination contains the following herbs: oak bark, marshmallow root, mullein herb, wormwood, lobelia, skullcap, comfrey root, walnut bark (or leaves) and gravel root.

Soak this herb combination in distilled water (at the rate of one ounce of combined herbs to a pint of distilled water), four to six hours, then simmer for thirty minutes, strain and reduce the liquid down to its volume by simmering over low heat. To retard spoilage of large batches, add vegetable glycerine. Example: One gallon of tea simmered (not boiled) down to two quarts and add one pint of glycerine.

Soak flannel, cotton or any natural material cloth in the solution-- never use synthetics. Wrap the fomentation (soaked cloth) around the malfunctioning area and cover with plastic to keep it from drying out. Leave on all night six nights a week, week after week, until relief appears.

Severe cases: Drink cup of finished concentrated tea with 3/4 cup of distilled water three times a day. (Also see formula No. 51.) Source: B F & C.

29. Hair Conditioner formula and procedure. To help restimulate hair growth, for two evenings massage scalp deeply with warm castor oil, apply hot, wet towel over head thirty minutes or more. Leave oil on all night. Next morning wash hair with pine tar soap or a good biodegradable soap and rinse. Wash again and rinse with tea made from this combination which contains; sagebrush, chaparral and yarrow. Massage well and leave tea in hair. The next two evenings do same procedure but use olive oil instead of castor oil and the next two evenings use wheat germ oil. Rest one night and repeat six days a week as needed. Use shoulder stands. Drink one or two tablespoons of wheat germ oil morning and night, and also drink cup of this tea made with distilled water, two times a day. Source: Desert Herb Combination.

30. Arthritis-Rheumatism formula. This combination consists of Brigham herb, hydrangea root, yucca, chaparral, lobelia, burdock root, sarsaparilla, wild lettuce, valerian, wormwood, cayenne, black cohosh, and black walnut. Here is a combination of herbs that detoxify; act as a solvent for the accepted but not assimilated calcium deposits; herbs that relieve pain; herbs rich in organic calcium that can be assimilated and useful; herbs that kill fungus and infection and give wonderful relief. This relief is not immediate because here is a long rebuilding job--gradual relief can come, and full healing, if the program is followed faithfully.

Take two capsules three times a day with a cup of Brigham tea or steam-distilled water. Use hot fomentations of this formula in tea form and formula No. 28 called bone, flesh, and cartilage over extremely painful or crippled areas. Also drink one or two quarts of kidney bean pod tea daily. In addition for relief, an external application of formula No. 44 is recommended. If one uses these aids yet continues with an improper diet, one may get some help but not as much. Remember the teachings for years have been--"No healing in this condition." We are giving you hope if you will follow through with these formulas and the mucusless diet. Sources: AR-1, Yucca AR.

31. Infection formula. This formula is made up of plantain, black walnut, golden seal root, bugle weed, marshmallow root and lobelia. This wonderful formula kills infection, clears toxins from the lymph system, and is a natural infection fighter. Dose 2 capsules three times a day or make a tea (empty 2 capsules into a cup and pour in boiling hot water). Sources: INF Combination, IF.

32. Kelp formula. This is an aid for the thyroid and assisting glands. These herbs assist in controlling metabolism and give herbal feeding to the thyroid glands to help them do their job more efficiently. This is a very fine glandular aid. The herbs combined are parsley, watercress, kelp, Irishmoss, romaine lettuce, turnip tops, Iceland moss. For additional help, use with formula No. 12. Source: Kelp-T, T Caps.

33. Antispasmodic tincture. Consists of skullcap herb, lobelia, cayenne, valerian root, skunk cabbage, myrrh gum and black cohosh. To be used in cases of convulsions, fainting, cramps, delirium, tremors, hysteria, etc., also good for pyorrhea, mouth sores, coughs, throat infections, tonsillitis, etc. Dose to one teaspoon to glass of steam distilled water as a gargle and use until throat clears, also take one teaspoon in steam distilled water morning and evening. Source: ANTSP.

34. B tincture. Consists of black cohosh, blue cohosh, blue vervain, skullcap, and lobelia. Used to aid in nervous conditions, sore throat, hiccups, restore malfunctioning motor nerves, assist in adjusting poor equilibrium and hearing, and a great blessing to epileptics. Massage into the medulla (base of skull), and upper cervicals, follow instructions in formula No. 14, and take six to ten drops in a little water or juice two or three times a day. Source: B&B.

35. Minor Pain Relief formula. This is a tincture or tea consisting of wild lettuce and valerian. It is to be taken orally or massaged externally as relief of minor pain. It is a natural sedative, quiet and soothing to the nerves. Source: Wild Lettuce & Valerian.

36. Asthma formula. An excellent asthma syrup--very helpful to expel mucus from the respiratory system. Can be used for sore throats and mucus. Excellent for fighting toxins. This is made of extracts of comfrey, mullein and garlic, and vegetable glycerine. Recommended use--a teaspoon or more, as required, as often as needed. Source: Comfrey-Mullein-Garlic syrup.

37. Cough formula syrup. A fine, old fashioned combination for coughs. Made up with fresh onion juice, licorice, honey and vegetable glycerine. Recommended use--a teaspoon or more, as required, as often as needed. Source: Herbal Cough.

38. Drawing ointment. For use externally on old ulcers, tumors, boils, warts, skin cancers, hemorrhoids, excellent for burns and as a healing agent. This is made with chaparral, comfrey, red clover blossoms, pine tar, mullein, beeswax, plantain, olive oil, mutton tallow, chickweed and poke root. Source: Black Ointment.

39. Healing ointment. Made of comfrey, marshmallow, marigold, bee's wax and oils, this is an antiseptic to be used on lesions, eczema, dry skin, poison ivy, abrasions, burns, hemorrhoids, bruises and swellings. Very soothing to inflamed surfaces. Good to have on hand at all times. Source: CMM.

40. Chickweed ointment. This is made of chickweed herb and bee's wax and oils. Excellent for eczema and/or other skin infections, sores, burning, itchy skin or genitals, swollen testes, acne, hives, also for ulceration of mouth and throat. This is a wonderful healing ointment. Source: Chickweed ointment.

41. Nose ointment. Made with spearmint, peppermint and vaseline, this is a natural anti-histamine. Apply to the inside of nose when it is congested, dry, sensitive or chapped. Source: Nose ointment.

42. Catnip and Fennel tincture. A blessing for infants. A fine combination for colic, teething pain, flatulence, spasms, etc. Use a few drops, or as much as needed when desired (available in alcohol and glycerine based extract). Source: Catnip & Fennel Tincture, Kid-E-Kol, Kol-X.

43. Black Walnut tincture. This is one of the best known remedies for fungus. Use externally and apply frequently. Source: Black Walnut tincture.

44. Cayenne salve. This penetrating salve contains olive oil, cayenne, oil of wintergreen, pure distilled mint crystals and other herb oils, in a beeswax base. It is excellent for stiff necks, sore muscles, headaches, pain, stiff joints, arthritis, etc. Source: Deep Heating Balm.

45. Antiseptic tincture. This is a wonderful first-aid tincture. Good for infection, both external or internal. The formula is: oak bark, golden seal root, myrrh, comfrey, garlic and capsicum, in a grain alcohol base. Source: X-Ceptic.

46. Heavy Mineral formula. Contains bugleweed, yellow dock, and lobelia. This is the herbal combination for combating pollution, both external and internal. It helps draw out minerals, drugs, and other pollutants trapped in our system. The dosage is two #0 capsules daily in conjunction with 6 #0 chaparral capsules taken three times a day. (This formula including the chaparral, is available in extract form.) Every other day bathe in 1 to 3 pounds of Epsom salts in a tub of hot water. The bathing routine should continue for three weeks then rest a week but continue taking the herbs. Source: Bugleweed combination.

47. Adrenals formula. Contains mullein, lobelia, Siberian ginseng, gotu kola, hawthorn berries, cayenne and ginger. As this formula corrects any imbalance in the adrenal glands it also compensates for any stress placed on the heart. Source: Adrenetone, ADR-NL.

48. Colitis formula. Contains marshmallow, slippery elm, comfrey root, lobelia, ginger and wild yam. This formula is for the relief of colitis, and should be used in conjunction with the lower bowel formula and the mucusless diet. Source: CC.

49. Ulcer formula. Contains bayberry, chickweed, slippery elm and mullein. This formula is designed to soothe the discomforts caused from stomach ulcers. It should be taken with hops or chamomile tea. Please note; to cure an ulcer, take three teaspoons of cayenne pepper

per day. This cayenne may be mixed in water or tomato juice. It is recommended that you start with only 1/8 teaspoon three times a day, then gradually work up to one teaspoon three time a day. Source: ULC.

50. Anti-Gas formula. Contains fennel, wild yam, catnip, ginger, peppermint, spearmint, papaya and lobelia. This formula was designed to relieve flatulence. Source: AT-GS.

51. Bone, Flesh and Cartilage ointment. Convenient form of formula No. 28. It is made into an ointment using an olive oil and beeswax base. Apply formula No. 41 after this for better penetration and quicker healing. Source: BF&C ointment.

52. Anti-Plague formula. The best remedy for colds, flu, or any communicable disease. This formula strengthens and stimulates your immune system and should be used as a tonic and preventative at the dosage of 1 tablespoon of syrup per day. If infected, the dosage changes to one tablespoon every hour. Anti plague syrup contains fresh garlic juice, apple cider vinegar, glycerine, honey, fresh comfrey root, wormwood, lobelia, marshmallow root, oak bark, black walnut bark, mullein leaf, skullcap and uva ursi. Source: ANT-PLG.

53. Cold Sore Relief formula. This formula, in extract form, is taken orally two droppers full 3 times a day and applied topically. Contents: fresh golden seal root, garlic and skullcap. Source: CSR.

54. Immune Stimulating formula -designed to enhance the body's ability to prevent the spread of bacteria and viruses. It consists of echinacea, calendula and red clover blossoms (available in alcohol extract or glycerine based extract for children). Sources: Imunacea, Kid-E-Mune, Immunaid.

55. Immune Calming formula -designed to calm yet strengthen the body's immune responses. Many times we believe that we are allergic to certain foods, plants or animals, but in reality our immune system may be just overreacting. This simple combination of marshmallow root and astragalus has made life easier for those who suffer from allergies, hayfever, asthma, rheumatoid arthritis or any hyperactive immune response. Sources: Imucalm, Kid-E-Soothe.

56. Memory formula -a great combination of old fashioned herbs used to cleanse and build and increase circulation to the brain. This formula consists of blue vervain, gotu kola, Brigham tea, ginko, blessed thistle, cayenne, ginger root, and lobelia. Source: MEM, REMEM.

57. Vitamin and Mineral formula -nature balanced, whole food vitamin and mineral supplement. This combination of alfalfa, dandelion, kelp, purple dulce, spirulina, Irish moss, rose hips, beet, nutritional yeast, cayenne, blue violet, oatstraw and ginger is an organic source of vitamins and minerals that are easy to assimilate because they are whole foods. Source: Vitalerbs.

58. Sinus Congestion formula. This very powerful formula consists of Brigham tea, horseradish, and cayenne. For immediate relief of sinus pressure due to cold or allergies, use 20 drops (teaspoon) in cup of hot water. May be taken every hour. Source: Ephedratean.

59. Rubefacient ointment. As the name indicates, this balm brings blood circulation to the surface of the skin causing it to turn red. Used to relieve tension and pressure. Great for tension headache or sinus pressure. Use sparingly as this formula is strong. Contains: olive oil and natural oils of cassia, eucalyptus, cajeput, pure menthol and camphor crystals and other fragrant natural oils. Source: Sen Sei balm.

60. Greens combination. A blend of alfalfa, barley grass and wheat grass herbs grown organically in virgin soil which is separated from urban and agricultural pollutants by the same mountains that provide its pure source of water. These herbs reduce acidity, provide needed chlorophyll and wholesome nutrients to the body.

61. Energy combination. Rather than being an energy jolt that shocks the body, this formulation of Siberian ginseng, bee pollen, licorice root, gotu kola, Brigham tea, yerba mate, and ginger root provides energy and vitality through wholesome nutrition.

PREPARATIONS

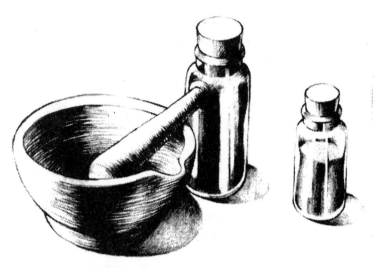

Vaginal herbal bolus:
To prepare a bolus, follow the instructions found with formula #24 in the formula section. Many women prefer to use unrefined olive oil instead of the coconut butter or oil as the base for the bolus but this requires cooling the olive oil till it is solid enough to mix with the herbs. Store them in the freezer till you are ready to use them. The bolus is self lubricating just by holding it in your hand till the oil melts over the surface of the bolus.

Capsules:
Purchase #0 or #00 capsules. Open and place inside the powdered herbs of your choice, tamping to fill completely. Close capsule.

Decoction:
Cover roots, barks, and other hard herbal material with water, an ounce of the herb to a pint and a half of water. Bring to a boil, and gently simmer for about twenty minutes to a half hour. Drain off the liquid while hot and press the herbs to make sure that the decoction is fully extracted. Decoctions are strong; take as directed.

Fomentation:

Soak a piece of gauze or a Turkish towel or similar porous material in the infusion or decoction needed. Sometimes hot apple cider vinegar is used. Cool until the material is just bearable for the patient. Cover with plastic or oilcloth to prevent the liquid from soaking bedclothes, etc. Keep damp and change periodically.

Infusion or Tea:

Pour boiling water over the herb, one teaspoonful of herb, cut, to the cup of water. Allow to steep fifteen to thirty minutes, strain, and give warm, sweetened with honey if desired.

Oil:

Crush the desired herb, bark, etc., and simmer in olive oil at 125-150° F. until the medicine comes out of the herb. This is often done in the oven. You can also make an oil by allowing the herb to sit in the oil in the direct sunlight for a week or more. Strain while hot. The proportions are about 1 to 4.

Ointments:

Make an herbal oil as above. Use about 4 tablespoons beeswax to the cup of oil. Melt both together, put into wide-mouthed container, and allow to cool without disturbing. Any of the soothing herbs make an excellent ointment, such as golden seal, slippery elm, marigolds, comfrey, cucumber, yarrow, meadowsweet, chickweed, wintergreen, eucalyptus, marshmallow root, mullein, etc. A variation that I use for plantain ointment: I blend the plantain directly into the olive oil until it's completely pulverized. Then I warm the pulpy oil until it can melt the beeswax and mix it all together. Let it harden as is. You'll get a green smear on your skin, but it's very healing. You can use lard as a base if you wish. Lard will not be absorbed into the body like the plant oils. Wheat germ oil can be added as part of the oil for its vitamin E content.

You can make a nice lip balm using these techniques which is better than lip ointments sold in stores. Make an oil using rose petals or marigold petals. Strain and warm, adding to the cup of rose oil, 1 tablespoon beeswax, 1 teaspoon honey, 1 teaspoon vanilla extract, 1 teaspoon wheat germ oil, and 1 teaspoon aloe vera gel. Warm and mix until thoroughly melted and pour into wide-mouthed, small containers.

(From Buchman's *Herbal Medicine*--an excellent book on herbal preparations and herb use generally.)

Tincture:

Take four ounces of crushed or chopped dry herbs or eight ounces of crushed fresh herbs. Cover with a quart of apple cider vinegar or 90-proof alcohol. Allow to steep for two weeks, shaking a few times each day. Strain out and label. Tinctures are given only by the drop; usually three or four drops can equal the dose of a cup of infusion of the same herb. Lobelia tincture is made in the vinegar, while other tinctures are often made in the alcohol.

For a glycerine tincture, which is good for non-oily or non-resinous herbs, soak the herbs in a pint of water and glycerine mixture-- 60% glycerine, 40% water. Proceed as above. Glycerine is available from vegetable sources, and it helps take toxins from the body.

Glycerine can also be added to a decoction or syrup to make it keep.

Syrup:

Most herbal syrups have a heavy sugary base, and I cannot recommend them. You can add a tincture to a spoonful of honey and take that for a syrup. Syrups are generally given to help children take herbs that might not in themselves be pleasant, or to soothe the throat.

Fluid Extract:

This herbal preparation is made commercially, but it is usually beyond the amateur herbal practitioner. You can use extracts as you do tinctures.

Electuary:

Add powdered herbs to syrup, honey, etc., to make a pleasant taste or easier administration.

Poultice:

Combine powdered or crushed herbs with enough slippery elm and hot water to make a thick paste. Put this over the affected area. A mustard poultice or plaster can help break up a heavy cough. Roasted onions can be crushed for the same purpose; they have been used in pneumonia. Raw grated onions will also work but you must coat the skin with olive oil beforehand and check for blistering consistently.

Wines:

You can use wine to make tincture, which is often more palatable to some. Diane Buchman suggests this tonic wine:

1	pint Madeira
1	sprig wormwood
1	sprig rosemary
1	small bruised nutmeg
1	inch bruised ginger root
1	inch bruised cinnamon bark
12	large organic raisins

Pour off about an ounce of the wine. Put the herbs in the wine. Cork the bottle and let macerate for a couple of weeks. Strain off, and combine this wine with a fresh bottle of Madeira, mixing thoroughly. Sip as needed during illness (*Herbal Medicine*, p. 218).

Tooth Powder:

Dr. Christopher suggested an herbal tooth powder that cleanses and heals the teeth and gums (see "Formulas," page 193). You can grind sage and sea salt together into a fine powder, drying in the oven, breaking it up or grinding it again if needed. This cleans off stains and tastes pleasant.

Breath Fresheners:

You can chew peppermint or spearmint leaves, fennel seeds, cloves (many times I saw Dr. Christopher chewing on a couple of cloves), mace, anise, and cinnamon for natural breath fresheners.

Lotion:

Homemade hand lotion is possible but not always easy to produce. Basically you are contriving a way to add water to oil and keep it there, for the oil can nourish the skin, but water moisturizes. Try this recipe:

Melt together
4	tablespoons lanolin

2   tablespoons coconut oil

3   tablespoons olive, safflower, or peanut oil

Pour these in a jar. Set aside.

In another container, mix:

2   tablespoons honey

1/4   cup lemon juice plus

1   tablespoon lemon juice

1/2   teaspoon lemon extract.

Add the second mixture to the first slowly, stirring constantly. Cap the jar and shake it until it cools and a lotion has formed. When the mixture is at room temperature (not before, or it will all curdle), whip in 3 tablespoons of water, using an electric mixer, one tablespoon at a time. Work patiently and slowly to incorporate all the water. Instead of lemon, you can use other fruits or herbs. Just blenderize the herbs, fresh if possible, or make a decoction, and strain. Use for the lemon part of the mixture. The lemon extract is just a scent, so you can add other herbal oils to scent the lotion as you desire. Refrigerate if you plan to keep it a long time.

Basic Lotion:

1   oz. lanolin or beeswax or coconut oil, or combination

3   fl. oz. natural oil, including 10 ml. wheat germ oil, if
         desired

2   fl. oz. of any herbal infusion, decoction, or flower
         water

3-6   drops of essential oil from any herb or flower

Melt the solid factor and add the oil, beating steadily, and then the water, added drop by drop. Take off the stove and stir until the mixture is at blood heat. Stir in the essential oil. Stir thoroughly and put into a pint bottle. Cap and shake until lotion is cool. Shake when using. The emulsion should hold.

Cream:

You can use any of the herbal ointments for face cream. Or try this recipe:

1   tablespoon beeswax
1   tablespoon olive oil
1   tablespoon lanolin
1   tablespoon liquid lecithin
3   tablespoons safflower or sunflower oil
2   tablespoons fresh unsalted butter

Melt this over hot water. Keep hot; watch carefully.

2 teaspoons glycerine
1/4 teaspoon borax (get at pharmacy)
1/3 cup water

Heat until it is at a simmer. Some people use a large electric skillet and set both pots in the hot water.
Now add the water mixture to the oil mixture slowly and carefully, beating with one beater on an electric beater. Keep beating until both mixtures combine completely. Stir until cool, off heat, and put in a clean, wide-mouthed jar. This is a very rich cream for dry skin, feels quite elegant.

Perfumes:

You might enjoy making herbal scents. You make an herbal oil as described above, using fresh blossoms, and straining out one batch and adding another until the scent becomes quite strong. An elegant way to make perfume is to put blossoms into a jar with just a bit of water in the bottom. The essential oil from the blossoms will collect on the water, and you can scrape off this scented oil and put it in tiny vials. Let the vial stand open for a couple of days to evaporate off any water. This essential scented oil is concentrated and very valuable. Use it to perfume other mixtures.

Herbal Steam:

Clean your face. Put two tablespoons of dried herbs or three handfuls of fresh herbs in a non-metal pot and pour over 3-1/2 pints boiling water. Stir. Tie your hair back. Hold your face about 8 inches from the pot and put a towel over your head to trap the steam.

Massage Oils:

Just add a few drops of essential oil, any of your favorites, to a natural oil, preferably olive.

REFERENCES

GENERAL

Buchman, Diane Dincin. Herbal Medicine. New York: Grammercy, 1980.

Christopher, John R. School of Natural Healing. Springville, Utah: Christopher Publications, 1976.

Christopher, John R. Herbal Home Health Care. Springville, Utah: Christopher Publications, 1978.

Grieve, Mrs. M. A Modern Herbal. New York: Dover, 1971.

Kloss, Jethro. Back to Eden. Loma Linda, California: Back to Eden Books, 1979.

Levy, Juliette de Bairacli-. Nature's Children. New York: Schocken, 1971.

Malstrom, Stan. Own Your Own Body. Bell Press, 1977.

Mendelsohn, Robert W. Male Practice. Chicago: Contemporary Books, 1981.

Meyer, David C. The Herbalist Almanac. Glenwood, IL: Meyerbooks, 1977.

Miller, Neil Z. Vaccines: Are They Really Safe and Effective?. Santa Fe, New Mexico: New Atlantean Press

Moore, Michael. Medicinal Plants of the Mountain West. Santa Fe, New Mexico: The University of New Mexico Press, 1979.

Mothering Magazine. P.O. Box 8410, Santa Fe, NM.

Parvati, Jeanine. Hygieia. A Woman's Herbal. Self-published, 1983.

Shook, Edward E. Advanced Treatise in Herbology. Beaumont, California: Trinity Center Press, 1979.

Tarr, Katherine. Herbs, Helps and Pressure Points for Pregnancy and Childbirth. Provo, Utah: Sunbeam Publications, 1984.

The People's Doctor. P.O. Box 982, Evanston, Illinoais 60204.

Tierra, Michael. The Way of Herbs. New York: Washington Square Press, 1983.

Weed, Susun S. Wise Woman Herbal, Childbearing Year. Woodstock: N Y.1985.

CHILDBIRTH AND PREGNANCY

Arms, Suzanne. Immaculate Deception. New York: Houton-Mifflin, 1973.

Baldwin, Rahima. Special Delivery. Millbrae, California: Les Femmes, 1979.

Block, Polly. Polly's Birth Book. American Fork, UT: Hearthspun Publishers, 1984.

Block, Polly. A Superior Alternative. Self-published, American Fork, UT,1979.

Bradley, Robert A. Husband-Coached Childbirth. New York: Harper and Row, 1975.

Eloesser, Leo, et.al. Pregnancy, Childbirth and the Newborn. Instituto Indigenista Interamicano, Mexico, 1973.

Garrey, Goven/Hodge/Callender, Obstetrics Illustrated. London: Churchill Livingstone, 1974.

Gaskin, Ina May. Spiritual Midwifery. Summertown, TN: The Book Publishing Company, 1978.

Gold, Cybele and E.J. Joyous Childbirth. Berkeley: And/Or Press, 1977.

Guay, Terrie. Avoid or Achieve Pregnancy Naturally. Emergence Publications, 1978.

Home Oriented Maternity Experience, Washington, D.C., 1976.

Karmel, Marjorie. Thank you, Dr. Lamaze. New York: Dolphin, 1975.

La Leche League. The Womanly Art of Breastfeeding, 1958.

"Midwifery and the Law," a *Mothering* Special Edition, Santa Fe, NM, 1990.

Moran, Marilyn A. Birth and the Dialogue of Love. Leawood, Kansas: New Nativity Press, 1981.

Patton, Joan. Midwifery, an unpublished course.

Practicing Midwife, The. 156 Drakes Lane, Summertown TB 38483.

Stewart, David and Lee. Safe Alternatives in Childbirth. Chapel Hill, NC: NAPSAC, 1976.

Wood, Camilla S., et.al. "Infant Nutrition, Communicating Nursing Research," Credibility in Nursing Science, Vol. 12:31-19, 1979 WICHEN.

Wright, Erna. The New Childbirth. New York: Pocket Books, 1967.

NUTRITION

Christopher, John R. Regenerative Diet. Springville, UT: Christopher Publications, 1982.

Littlegreen Inc.'s Think Tank. Transfiguration Diet. 1986. Christopher Publications Springville, UT

Nutrition Almanac. New York: McGraw Hill, 1973

Tracy, Michael. The Mild Food Cookbook, Christopher Publications Springville, UT

Wigmore, Ann. Be Your Own Doctor. Wayne, New Jersey: Avery, 1982

COSMETICS

Little, Kathy. Book of Herbal Beauty. New York: Penguin, 1980.

Traven, Beatrice. The Complete Book of Natural Cosmetics. New York: Simon & Schuster, 1974.

INDEX

Entries in full capital letters indicate either a formulation name or a section heading.

A

ABO blood
   incompatibility 94
abortifacient 4
abortion I, 3, 4, 16, 17,
   20, 31, 44
Abscessed Tooth 158
abuse 149
abusive language 113
accupressure 76, 153
acid balance 156
acidity 155
acidophilus 92, 93, 152,
   166
acne 1, 6, 7
activated charcoal 38
additives 147
adoption, anecdote 88
ADR-NL 201
adrenal glands 133, 201
Adrenals formula 201
Adrenetone 201
aerobics 141
AFTERPAINS 81
AIDS epidemic 107
Alaska 26, 127
alcohol 80, 128, 156, 188
alfalfa 27, 203
allergic reaction 145
allergies 99, 156, 203
   food 97,145
allergies, sinus, and
   hayfever formula 157,
   190
allergy headaches 145
almonds 133
Aloe vera 81, 84, 166
aluminum ware 140
Alzheimer's disease 154

amniocentesis 31
amphetamines 127
amputation 131
anemia 38
   anecdote 109
anesthesia 55
ANT-PLG 202
antacids 38
anti-depressants 127
anti-gas formula 124,
   202
anti-histamine 200
Anti-Miscarriage formula
   197
Anti-Obese Herbal Food
   formula 191
anti-plague formula 120,
   202
antibiotic 101, 155
antihistamine 157, 190
antiseptic tincture 92,
   138, 201
antispasmodic tincture
   161, 199
ANTSP 199
Appendicitis 158
appendix 159
apple cider vinegar 156,
   166
   and honey mixture 143
Apple juice 6, 121
AR-1 199
arthritis 143, 203
   of the spine 117
Arthritis-Rheumatism
   formula 198
Aspirin 13
asthma 8, 124, 192, 203
asthma formula 126, 200

astragalus 203
astringents 7
AT-GS 202
avocado 181

B

B F & C 10, 198 (see
  bone, flesh...)
B tincture 103, 135, 199
B&B 192, 199
B-vitamin 38, 43, 46
B/P 191
BABY CLOTHES 68
baby food, grinding 91
baby, giving herbs to 94
  need to live quietly. 96
  oil preparation 100
  powder 99
  premature 100
  slings 96
  tense 80
baby's blood glucose 87
baby's spirit 108
baby-sitters 22
Bach Rescue Remedy
  69,81
BACKACHE 39
barberry 187
Barberry LG 188
barefoot V
barley leaves 28
Basil 2
bath 2, 39, 83, 103, 150
bayberry 164, 193, 194
beans 25
Bed Wetting formula 188
behavior, criminal 148
Bendectin 29
Berberis vulgaris 185
berries 26

BF&C ointment 202
bilirubin 93
bilirubin lights 94
Billings, John and Evelyn
  1 8
birth 197
  drugged 55
  low birth weight 54
birth control 13,15, 17,
  52 the Pill 16
birth day 65
birth defects 154
BIRTH INJURES 54
birthing bed 67
Birthing centers 50
birthing position 58
biting bugs 163
black cohosh 43, 192,
  1 9 9
Black Ointment 200
black walnut 100, 152
Black walnut tincture
  122, 163, 164, 201
bleed overmuch 80
blessed thistle 2, 43, 88,
  89, 90, 203
blind 129
blood cleansing formula
  133 (see blood purify..)
blood clots 197
blood poisoning 105
blood pressure 156
blood pressure formula
  43, 190
blood purifying formula
  133, 172, 187
blood stream 187
blood sugar 87, 150
blue cohosh 81, 192, 199

blue vervain 199, 203
blue violet 203
body temperature 168
boils 200
bolus 196
BONE CANCER 116
bone, broken 120, 159
bone, flesh, and cartilage
  143, 160, 165, 197
  fomentation 9, 198, 114
  ointment 202 recipe 9
botulism in honey 93
bowel movement 139
bowel pocket 123
BPE 191
Bradley method 77
brain 203
bread 178 (also see pita)
BREAST CANCER 118
BREAST INFECTION 83
  anecdote 110, 111
breast milk (also see
  mother's milk) 90
  for eye infection 86
breast milk jaundice 94
breastfeeding 86, 88, 91,
  99 (also see nursing)
breath freshener 207
Breathe-Aid 193
breathing V
breech 74
brewer's yeast 90, 101,
  151
Brigham tea 124, 157,
  190, 203
Bright's Disease 132
Broken Bones 120, 161
bronchials 192
bronchitis 192

bruises 136, 159
Buchman, Diane 207
bug biting 163
bugleweed 129, 199, 201
Bugleweed combination
  201
Burdock 6, 165
burn paste 159, 166
burns 159

C

C&F 193
C-complex 41
C-section (see Caesarean)
CA-T 190
Caesarean section 48, 53,
  56, 74, 111
cajeput 203
Calc Tea 190
calcium 42, 46, 82, 142,
  164, 166
calcium deposits 198
calcium formula 39, 40,
  42, 46, 143, 145, 166,
  190 recipe 83
calcium imbalance 83
calcium spurs 197
Calctean 190
camphor 203
cancer 15, 16, 26, 32, 52,
  58, 114, 116, 118
cancer, breast 115, 168
cancer of the cervix 119
candidias albicans 41,
  152, 157
Capsicum fastigiatum 185
Capsicum minimum 185
Capsules 204
cardiac tonic 189
cardiovascular disease

153
career 169
caretaker IV
Carrot juice 6, 46, 118,
    171
casein 86
casseroles 176
castor oil 48, 64, 135
cataracts 130, 153
Catnip 2, 80, 93, 98, 159
catnip and fennel
    tincture 98, 201
catnip enema 102,144
cayenne 12, 43, 57, 81,
    130, 131, 153, 162,
    164, 172, 189, 190,
    193, 194
cayenne in eye 131
cayenne ointment, salve
    12, 146, 161,201
cayenne tincture 82
CC formula 202
cedar berry 132
celery juice 133, 147
cell proliferant 27
cervix 66
    herbs to loosen 76
Change-O-Life 196
Changease 43, 196
chaparral 198
charlie horse 190
cheese 26, 145
chamomile VII, 102, 130,
    136, 150, 166
chemicals 152, 156
chemotherapy 115
chewing food 157 162
chia seeds 37, 133
    sprouts 177

chickweed 86, 163, 191
    ointment 200
chiropractor 39, 92, 98,
    144
chlamydial infection 85
chorion biopsy 33
cigarettes 128
CIRCUMCISION 97
Circutean 191
civilization 127
clamp, umbilical 79
classical music 141
cleanliness 55
cleansing 47 crisis 184
Clomid 20
clothing 147
cloves 166, 193
CMM ointment 200
cobbler 183
cocaine 127
coffee 128, 188
Cold Sore Relief 202
Cold Sores 161
colds 101, 193, 202
colic 90, 91, 97, 194, 201
    bath remedy 99 dill-
    water treatment 98
Colitis formula 202
college III
Collins, Cardiss 127
comfrey 81, 93, 159, 161,
    193, 197
comfrey combination 197
comfrey paste 117
comfrey tea 120
Comfrey-Mullein-Garlic
    syrup 200
Composition formula 193
computers 154

congestion 124
CONJUNCTIVITIS 86
CONSTANT CONTACT 95
constipated warriors 138
CONSTIPATION 37, 138
  headache, 144
contraction, stimulate 80
convulsions 87, 161, 164
cooked food 173
cord around the neck 79
cord clamp 67
cord stump 79 alcohol 80
cost, mucusless diet. 183
cotton 153
cough 101, 161, 206
Cough formula syrup 200
counseling 148
cow's milk 86
cradle cap 100
cramping 164
cranberry juice 155
Crataegus oxycantha 189
cravings 26, 128, 184
Cream recipe 208
criminal behavior 148
crooked teeth 190
croup 161
CSK Plus 191
CSR 202
cucumber 43
curvature, spine 117, 197
cuts 159
cycles (see menstruation)
cysts 14, 111, 122, 196
CYSTS AND TUMORS 121

D

D&C 52
dairy 97, 99, 145
dandelion 37, 93, 94, 163

DEAFNESS, EAR
  TROUBLES 135
decoction 204
decongestant 190
Deep Heating Balm 12,
  39, 82, 146, 165, 201
deformed 114
dehydration 101,103,
  146, 166
  treatment for Babies
  102
Delalutin 21
delivery, anecdote 58
Demerol 55
descending colon 123
Desert Herb Combination
  198
Desserts 182
DIABETES 132, 153
diagnosis 144 (also see
  reflexology)
diaper rash 92, 99
diaphoretic herbs 102
diaphragm 17
diarrhea 91, 103
diet 30, 115, 191, 141
diet pill 126
digestion 143, 162
  vinegar for 172
digestive system,
  immature 97
dilation, 56, 77 self
  check 66
dill 162 for colic 98
diphtheria 105
distilled water 48, 90,
  110, 117
dong quai 80
Doppler stethoscope 33

douche, herbs used 153
Down's syndrome 31
DPT vaccine 104
drawing ointment 200
dreams 147, 149
DRI 188
drink your solids 162
DRUG ABUSE 126
drugged birth 55
drugs 55, 73, 147
  heavy 128
  illicit 127
  jaundice occurs 93
  steroid 124
DRY SKIN, CRADLE CAP
  100
dulse 172
dysmenorrhea 2
dyspnoea 189

E

EAR INFECTION 103
ear syringe 67
earaches 136, 161
early nursing 75, 87
ear scope 104
echinacea 65, 101, 153,
  155, 202
Echinacea and garlic 83
eczema 200
edema 132
elder flower 102
elderberry tincture 122
electuary 206
eliminative channels 172
EMOTIONAL HEALTH 146
emotional stress 28
emotions 55, 147
emphysema 192
employed III

encephalitis 106
enema 103, 139
  garlic enema 102
energy 184
ENERGY-GIVING HERBS
  76
ENGORGEMENT 82
environment 55
Ephedratean 203
ephedrine 124
epileptic 136, 199
episiotomy 73 rate in
  hospital 53
Epsom salts 201
equilibrium 192, 199
eruptive diseases 161
estrogen 2, 43, 168, 195
  breast cancer link 168
estrogen pills 168
eucalyptus 203
Ex-Stress 192
EXCLUSIVE
  BREASTFEEDING 87
exercise 34, 133, 146,
  148, 153
exercise program 141
EXPELLING THE
  PLACENTA 80
eye, foreign particle in
  162
eye infection 86
eye reading (see
  iridology)
eye teeth 91
eye troubles 162
eyebright 86, 194
eyebright formula 129
eyestrain 154
eyewash formula 194

recipe 130

F

fainting 199
faith 51, 149
false labor 66
false unicorn 197
false unicorn and lobelia
combination 21, 43, 197
false unicorn root 195
family 22, 146, 148
family bed 96
Farm, The 53
FEM 195
female corrective formula
13, 48, 109-111,151,
169, 194
Fematean 196
FEN LB 187
fennel 193, 202
fertility 13, 18, 21
fertility drug 20, 21
fetal monitoring 56
fetal stethoscope. 33
fetoscopy 33
FEVER 101
teething. 102
bath remedy for 103
feverfew tea 145
fiber, natural 147
finger, cut off 10, 160
flatulence 201, 202
flour 152, 156, 173
flu 101, 119, 194, 202
bath remedy 103
flu shots 106
fluid extract 206
Foeniculum vulgaris 186
folic acid 38
follicular stimulating

hormone 168
fomentation 205
food allergies 97
food, gas-forming 97
Foote, Loretta 49
forceps 55 in hospital 53
FORMULA (for baby) 86
FORMULAS, herbal 185
fragarine 27
Frantz, Kitty 108
fruits 173
fungus 163, 198

G

GALLSTONES 121
GANGRENE I, 131, 132
garbage collectors 106
garden 169
Garlic 43, 65, 92, 101,
152, 155, 156, 163, 191
douche 153 enema 102,
167 extract in oil 99,
103, 135 juice 158, 202
Garlic, Rosehips &
Parsley 193
gas 38, 90, 123,
162 (see flatulence)
Gatorade, substitute 77
Gazpacho 181
German measles vaccine
106
ginger 2, 12, 27, 76, 145,
167, 190, 193, 202
ginger ale 28
ginger bath 145
ginko 203
ginseng 43, 76, 166, 195
glands 191
glaucoma 130
glycerite 94 tincture 206

goat's milk 88
God 116
golden seal 68, 79, 86, 194, 199, 202
  douche 153
gonorrheal blindness 85
gout 143
grains, preparation 173
gratitude 78
gravel root 195, 197
green drink 6, 8, 27, 29, 82, 161
Greenwood, Sadja 170
growth spurts 90
gums 137

H

Hair Conditioner 198
HAIR LOSS 134
halvah 177
Hannah and Samuel 91
hard water 188
HAS 190
hawthorn berries 43, 133, 156, 191
hawthorn berry syrup 162, 189
hayfever 157, 203
HEADACHES 144-146
  allergy related 145
healing ointment 200
health, perfect V
hearing 136, 199
Hearing Loss and Earache formula 192
heart attack 123, 156, 162
HEART DISEASE 156
Heart formula 189
heartburn 38

Heavy Mineral formula 201
hemorrhage 80
hemorrhoids 40, 196, 200
Hepatean 188
HERBAL FORMULAS 171
Herbal Bolus formula 196
Herbal Cleanse 110, 111, 117, 171
Herbal Composition 194
Herbal Cough 200
Herbal Eyebright 194
herbal first aid 158
Herbal L.B 187
herbal steam 209
Herbal Tooth Powder 193
herbs for: colic 98
  constipation 140
  drug detoxification 129
  ear troubles 136
  eye problems 130
  gangrene 132
  gums 138
  hair growth 135
  headaches 146
  heart 156
  labor 64, 69, 76
  losing weight 142
  poisonings 164
  teeth 138
heroin 127
hiccups 199
HIGH BLOOD PRESSURE 43, 153 in hospital 53
high blood sugar 132
high risk home birth 52
high-risk pregnancy 33
HIV 107
hoarseness 194

holy thistle 195, 197
HOME BIRTH, HIGH RISK
  FOR 50
home birth 57, 75, 112
  advantages of 58
honey 93, 159
hops 192
hormonal imbalance 143
hormone balancing
  formula 13, 43, 48, 88,
  109-111, 151, 169, 195
HORMONES 43, 2, 168
horseradish 190, 203
horsetail grass 46, 155,
  193
hospital births 54
hospitals, true use 92
hot flashes 169
houndstongue 165
Hoxey 187
hunger, hidden , 2
husband to catch baby 79
hydrangea root 198
Hydrastis canadensis 186
hydrochloric acid 143,
  156
hydrogenated oil 7, 25
hydrophobia 162
hyperactive immune
  response 203
hypertrophy 189
hypoglycemia 87, 132
hypothalamus gland 168
hyssop 164
hysterectomies 109
hysteria 199

I

IF 199
Immunaid 203

Immune Calming formula
  203
Immune Stimulating
  formula 202
immune system 101, 107
  157
immunity 91
IMMUNIZATIONS 104,
  107, 108
immunologic response
  105, 107
immunosuppressor 107
Imucalm 203
Imunacea 203
INAPPSAC, the 64
incontinence 111, 188
INCURABLES 112
Incurables Program 9,
  113, 114, 117
  anecdote 112
INDIGESTION 38, 162
  chronic 163
induce labor 64
INF Combination 199
infant botulism 93
Infant death rate 54
infection 101, 155, 158
  bladder VI; breast 83;
  chlamydial 85; ear 103;
  eye 86; gum 136;
  ovaries 110; skin 10;
  urinary 41; yeast 41,
  92, 99, 124
Infection formula 199
influenza 101, 119
infusion 205
insect bites 162-163
insect repellent 23, 163
insect stings 163

INSOMNIA 150, 192
  anecdote 150
insulin 132, 189
interaction 127
internal exams 56
intestinal flora 91, 143
Intestinal Parasites
  formula 193
intuition 108
  to choose midwife 64
iridology 110, 113, 144
iron 27
irritability 150, 152
itching 11, 163
  skin 41, 200
IUD 16, 52

J

jaundice 52, 93
  pathological 94
Jerusalem artichokes 133
Journal of Reproductive
  Medicine, The 54
juice after birth 69
Juni-Pars 188
juniper berries 155
Juniperas monostone 132
junk food 7, 26
Jurassic Green 46

K

KB formula 188
Kegel exercises 35
kelp 172, 203
Kelp formula 199
Kid-E-Calc 190
Kid-E-Kol 201
Kid-E-Mune 203
Kid-E-Soothe 203
Kidney and Bladder
  formula 110, 172, 188

kidneys 39, 188
kinesiology 92
knee 160
Kol-X 201

L

La Leche League 87
LABOR 65, 70
  anecdote 57, 72, 78
laborade, 77
LABOR HERBS 69, 64, 76,
  for pain 78
Lamaze breathing 77
lambsquarters 38
language, abusive 113
lanolin 83
laxatives 37, 139
Leboyer method 80
lecithin 156, 209
leeches 122
leg, broken 120
  stiff 160
legality of home birth 59
lemon juice 155
lemonade 162
lentil-rice casserole 176
lesions 200
leukemia 153
LG formula 188
Librium 127
lice 164
licorice 2, 43, 133, 191
Liedloff, Jean 95
linseed 163
lip balm 205
live food 116
live-polio vaccine 105
liver, damaged 94
  to combat cancer 118

liver-gall bladder
formula 110, 118, 172, 187
lobelia 8, 76, 98, 103, 125, 136, 158, 161, 185, 197, 199
for labor pain 78
for shock 81
lobelia tincture 82, 206
lochia 82
lockjaw 105
lotion 207
lovemaking during pregnancy 30
premature 6
low blood sugar 132
lower bowel formula 37, 49, 110, 111, 117, 133, 144, 151, 172, 185,
Lower Bowel Tonic 7, 128, 152 anecdote 139 (also see lower bowel formula)
Lungs and Respiratory Tract formula 126, 192
lupus 107
lymph system 199

M

malefern 193
Malfunctioning Glands formula 191
malnutrition 127
and tetanus 105
malpositioned 51
margarine 7, 25
marigold 200
marijuana 4, 127
marshmallow 90, 131, 203

massage 76, 146, 150
baby 102, 103
castor oil 198
perineum 73
massage oils 210
mastitis 89, 191
MATERNAL DEATH RATE 54
mayonnaise 175
measles vaccination 106
meat 26, 145
meconium 68, 93
medical care 125
medical intervention 156
medical profession 49
meditation 142, 146, 148
Mehl, Lewis, et al. 54
MEM formula 203
Memory formula 203
Mendelsohn, Robert MD 32, 109, 127
menstrual cramps 2, 12, 164
menstrual pads 3
menstruation 1, 109
irregular 23, 194
mental institution 150
midwife 49
intuition to choose 64
midwifery 59
migraine headache 144-145
milk 156, 180
Milk thistle seed 94
mind, frame of 117
mind-altering drugs 127
mineral oil 99
minerals 142
mint crystals 201

MISCARRIAGE 44, 154
  recurring 43
mistletoe 81
mistreatment, doctor 109
molasses 173
moles 122
monkey virus 107
mono diets 155
moon 23
morning sickness 27
mother's milk 87, 88
motherwort 42, 78, 81
motion sickness 167
motor nerve 192, 199
mucus 192, 200
  slippery elm to cut 91
mucusless diet 2, 6, 90,
  121, 141, 152, 171, 172
mullein 136
mullein and lobelia 159,
  191
mullein oil 136, 161
multiple sclerosis 15,
  107, 119
mumps vaccine 106
muscle, cramped 164
  pulled 197
MUSCLE PAINS 39
mustard poultice 206
myrrh 68, 79, 158, 199

N

natural birth (see birth)
Naturalax "2" 187
near-sighted 130
neck, stiff 165
nerve herbal food formula
  147, 150, 192
nerve sheath 190, 192
Nervean 192

nervousness 147, 192
neurological illness 104
neurosis 188
newborn 85
nightmares 164
nipples, sore 83
non-stress test 33
Nose ointment 200
nosebleed 164
Nowell, Dr. 193
Nu Fem 195
nursing 75, 80, 87,
  anecdote 89
  contracts uterus 80
  for comfort 90
  give herbs while 101
  how long to 90
  how often to 89
  to keep milk down 103
  prolonged 91
  (also see breastfeeding)
nut loaf 182
nut milk 180
nutritional yeast 203
nylon stockings 3

O

oak bark 40, 100, 137,
  167, 193
oil preparations 205
oil of cloves 102
oil of garlic 135, 192
oil of mullein and lobelia
  103
oil of rosemary 100
ointments 205
  healing 200
okra 163
Old Testament 91
olive oil 7, 48, 67, 73,

100, 121, 135, 146, 152
olive oil massage 100
onion juice 158, 200
onion syrup 161
onions 152, 161
operation, cost 121
oracles 169
orange juice 162
Os, not fully dilated, 78
OSTEOPOROSIS 142
Ott, John 154
out of doors 127
ovaries 168
   with infection 110
overdue 65
overweight 52, 140
Ovulation Method 18
oxytocin 73
   use in hospital 53

P

Pancratean 190
PAIN 77, 192
   in menstruation 2, 14
   in the ovaries 111
Pain Relief formula 200
Panc Tea 190
pancreas 132, 143
pancreas formula 133,
   143, 157, 189
papaya 191
Paprika 46
pau d'arco 152
PC formula 190
peanut butter 7
Pedialyte solution 77
pelvic rock 36
pelvis, broken 160
   immature 113
penicillin 85

peppermint 8, 12, 98,
   102, 125, 145
peppermint/lobelia
   treatment 124
perfume 209
PERINEAL HYGIENE 81
peristaltic muscles 186
pertussis vaccine 104
petroleum-based oil 99
phlegm 125
phosphorus 142
phototherapy 94
physiological jaundice 93
pine tar soap 198
pinkeye 86
pinto beans 134
pita 179
placenta 72, 80
Placydil tranquilizer 127
plantain 94, 105, 199
   ointment 165
   poultice 162
PMS 151
PN-6 197
pneumonia 92, 101, 206
   vaccine 106
poison 162
poison ivy. 165
poison oak 165
poisons 164
polio 9
   vaccination 105, 107
pollen 157
pollution 127, 147, 166
poplar bark 163
potassium 134
   broth 122, 181
poultice preparation 206
power drink 134

PR formula 195
prayer 51, 115, 142, 146
pre-natal formula 74
Pre-Natal Tea 197
Prednisone 13, 124
pregnancy formula 27
premature babies 100
prenatal deaths 53
PRENATAL FORMULA 67, 76, 197
prenatal nutrition 25
PREPARATORY LABOR 66
preservatives 147
processed food 147
progesterone 43
Prolapsed Organ formula 196
prolapsed, colon 110
uterus, bowel, 196
Prospallate 195
prostate formula 195
protein 25, 42, 176, high quality sources 133
Provera 21
prune juice 6
psoriasis 9
psychiatrist 148
psychological therapy 148
puberty 1
pudding 183
pumpkin seeds 167
puncture wound 105, 165
pushing 79
PYORRHEA (INFECTION OF THE GUMS) 136, 193

Q

queen of meadow root 195

R

R.C.C. 187
radiation 153
radical mastectomy 118
radish sprouts 178
rape 20
R.E.M. sleep 147
raspberry (see red rasp.)
RECIPES 175
    B.F. & C. formula 9
    bread, sprouted 178
    burn paste 117
    calcium formula 83
    cream 208
    eyewash formula 130
    Gazpacho 181
    ginger ale 28
    headache remedy 145
    insect repellent 163
    laborade, 77
    lemonade 162
    lentil casserole 176
    lotion 207
    mayonnaise 175
    nut milk 180
    onion syrup 161
    power drink 134
    pudding 183
    salad bar 175
    seed candy 177
    shock tea 57
    smoothie 174
    sauce, white 182
    stress remedy 145
red clover 6
red clover combination 110, 128, 152, 187
red clover sprouts 178
red raspberry 12, 13, 48, 90, 92, 110, 161, 162,

194
REFLEXOLOGY 71, 72, 76, 123, 144, 145
refried beans 25
Rejuvelac 143, 178
Relax-Eze 192
religious belief 78
REM 147
REMEM 203
Renatean 188
REPRODUCTIVE SYSTEM 110, 194
Rescue Remedy 165
Resp-Free 193
respiratory therapy 125
responsibility 148
Respratean 193
rest on seventh day 172
RH FACTOR 48
Rh-negative problem 51
Rhamnus purshiana 185
Rheum palmatum 186
ringing in ears 136
rite of passage 169
RNA and proviruses 107
rock music 141
rose hips 83, 166, 193, 203
rose oil 205
rosemary 193
Rothman, Barbara Katz 31
rouleaux 154
Rubefacient ointment 203
Rubus idaeus 186
ruptured membrane 56

S

sagebrush 198
salad bar 175
salt 42

sarsaparilla 2, 43, 198
sauce, white 182
scabs 11
scar tissue 49, 111
scream 79
Seconal 55
sedatives 126
seed candy 177
seeds, sprouting 177
SELF-EXAM 66
self-reliance 95
Sen Sei balm 203
SERIOUS ILLNESS 91
sesame seed 46, 178
sexual drive 170
sexual intercourse 20, 21
sexual intimacy 5
SHA Tea 190
shepherd's purse 81
shock 57, 165
  lobelia for 81
shock tea 57,69, 76, 81, 165 anecdote 72
shots 104
SIDS (see Sudden Infant Death Syndrome)
silica 46, 142, 190
SILVER NITRATE 85
sinus congestion formula 157, 203
sinus pressure 203
Sinutean 190
sitz bath 34, 39, 40
skin 147
  disease 9
  dry 100
  eruptions 197
  infection 10
skullcap 78, 192, 199

skunk cabbage 199
slant board 196, 110, 152
slippery elm 38, 100,
    103, 159, 202
  gruel 91, 98
SLM 191
Smallpox vaccination 106
snake bite 162
soak 10, 103, 131
soap 7
soft drinks 156, 188
sore throat 200
soup 184
soy milk 180
spider cancer 15
spine 118, 192
  deteriorated 117
sprains 165, 197
sprouts 184
  bread 178
  milk 180
St. John's Wort 78
stamina 168
state law on midwifery 59
statistics of hospital and
  home births 53
steam-distilled (see
  distilled water)
sterilize, how to 67
steroid drugs 124
stomach teeth 91
stomach flu 119
stomach ulcers 202
stones 111, 121
strawberries 8
strawberry barley
  pudding 183
streptococcus from
  vaccine 104

stress 127, 133, 145,
    152, 154
stroke 153
styptic 81
suburb 146
Sudden Infant Death
  Syndrome 91, 104
sugar 99, 144, 147, 153,
    155, 156, 181
sugar headache 144
suicide 9
summer soup 181
sunbathe 112, 135
sunburn 166
sunflower seeds 133
sunlight and bilirubin 93
  and diaper rash 99
SUPPLIES FOR HOME
  BIRTH 67
surgery 13
  unnecessary 73
sweeteners 181
swimming 34, 118
synthetics 4, 68, 147
syrup preparation 206
            T
T Caps 199
talcum powder 99
tea, preparation 205
tear duct, plugged 86
TECHNOLOGY 153
teeth, first 91 eye 91
  loose 137
TEETHING 102
  bath remedy for 103
tension 12, 40, 97, 127
tension headache 203
tetanus 165
  caused by diet 105

Tetracycline 85
The Farm 53
The Inter-National Association of Parents and Professionals for Safe Alternatives in Childbirth 64
The Journal of Reproductive Medicine, 54
Theophylline 124
thievery, 96
three-day cleanse 6, 111-112, 121, 128, 171
three-oil massage 48, 110, 112 **135**
thrombosis 16
thrush 92
thymus gland 107
thyroid 173, 199
  cancer 153
  malfunction 191
tinctures 69
  lobelia 103
  preparation 206
tobacco 156
tonsillitis 199
tooth ache 138, 166
  decay 138
Tooth Powder formula 193, 207
TOXEMIA 42
trace minerals 143, 173
Tracy, Michael 183
tranquilizers 126, 147
travel 166
tremors 197
tuberculosis 192
tumors 14, 111, 121, 196

Tylenol 13

U

ULC 202
Ulcer formula 202
ultrasound 32, 56
umbilical cord (see cord)
urethral canal 188
URINARY INFECTION 41, 155
uterus removed 110
  underdeveloped 113
Uva ursi 155, 195

V

vaccination, effect of 107
  cases among household contacts 106
  (also see immunization and "type of"-vaccine)
V.B. 196
vaginal birth after Caesarean 74
  bolus 109-111
  drainage 110
  irritation 153
Valerian 145, 150, 161, 192, 200
Valium 127
Vanceril 124
varicose veins 40, 167, 197
VBAC 74, 112
vermicide 193
vermifuge 193
vernix 59
vertebrae, missing 117
VF Syrup 193
vibrations 147
video display terminals

154
violet leaves 37
Virginia snake root 76
viruses 107, 202 (see
 infection)
VISION TROUBLES 129
Vitalerbs 203
vitamin A 38
vitamin B 151, 173
vitamin B-"12" 46
vitamin B-"6" 27, 87
vitamin C 22, 45, 83, 151,
 156
vitamin C-complex 41
Vitamin and Mineral
 formula 203
vitamin E 21, 37, 45, 135,
 173, 205
vitamin K 27
VITAMINS 45, 6
VOMITING 103

W

walk 12, 127, 150
 helps colic 98
walnut leaves 164
warts 122, 200
water 145
wean 90
weaning feast 91
 food 91
weariness 152
weave 169
weight 191
WEIGHT GAIN 30
weight problem 10, 141
wheat 151
wheat bread 179
wheat germ oil 48, 135,
 156, 159, 162, 166,

173, 198
wheat grass 166
wheat grass juice 39, 94,
 159
wheelchair 114, 119
wheezing 125
Wigmore, Ann 178, 184
white oak (see oak)
white sauce 182
white flour 99
whooping cough 104
wild lettuce 200
Wild Lettuce & Valerian
 200
wild yam 17, 64, 123,
 124, 202
wine preparation 207
wormwood 193
wound 165

X

X-Ceptic 201
X-rays 33, 153

Y

yarrow 155, 198
yeast infection 41, 99,
 124,
 vaginal 152
YEAST INFECTION IN
 BABIES 92
yellow dock 37, 109, 129,
 196, 201
Yellow Dock Combination
 37, 197
yucca 198
Yucca AR 199

Z

Zingiber officinale 185
zone therapy 71
zucchini 8

Additional Titles by Dr. John R. Christopher

DR. CHRISTOPHER'S HERBAL SEMINAR VIDEOS (9 VHS or PAL tapes) Over 16 hours of Dr. Christopher on video cassette. Witness America's premier natural healer sharing the knowledge and simple techniques gained from over 30 years of very successful herbal practice. Tape 1 $40.00 - Tapes 2-5 $160.00 - Tapes 6-9 $160.00

SCHOOL OF NATURAL HEALING The reference volume of natural healing for the teacher, student or herbal practitioner. Over 700 pages of instruction on the use, action, description, application and formulation of herbs. This knowledge comes to you from Dr. Christopher's experience of over 30 years of successful herbal practice. $39.95

DR. CHRISTOPHER'S NEW HERB LECTURES (10 cassette tapes - 1 hour each) Listen and glean from the knowledge, wit and wisdom of Dr. Christopher teaching the benefits of herbs and natural healing. Special mind trac summaries at the end of each tape will aid the student to retain this vital information. $69.95 (includes 2 bonus tapes)

HERBAL HOME HEALTH CARE This work from Dr. Christopher effectively deals with over 50 common ailments, listing the diseases in convenient alphabetical order with concise definitions, symptom descriptions, causes, herbal aids and other natural treatments, 196 pages. $12.95

REGENERATIVE DIET Dr. Christopher's herbal diet plan for healthy living. Includes menu plans with nutritional analysis. 275 pages. $7.95

CAPSICUM Dr. Christopher's research and case histories detailing the uses and healing powers of cayenne pepper. This herbal work is HOT! 166 pages. $6.95

New Release -DR. JOHN R. CHRISTOPHER: AN HERBAL LEGACY OF COURAGE The first biography of Dr. Christopher. Learn about his youth, his roots in herbalism, and his joys and struggles as he sought to heal and educate all who would hear. $5.00

Continued on next page...

DR. CHRISTOPHER'S THREE DAY CLEANSE, MUCUSLESS DIET AND HERBAL COMBINATIONS Juice and herbal cleansing, wholesome diet plan, herb formulas, simple therapies, and more. $2.00

REJUVENATION THROUGH ELIMINATION Dr. Christopher goes into detail on his lower bowel formula and even gives the recipe. Excellent discussion on cleansing and nourishing the bowel to obtain a disease free body. $2.00

THE INCURABLES Complete, wholistic, treatment program for conditions deemed "incurable." Dr. Christopher shows "there are no incurable diseases." $2.00

THE COLD SHEET TREATMENT Dr. Christopher explains step by step, his time tested treatment for colds, flu and any feverous or viral condition. $1.75

JUST WHAT IS THE WORD OF WISDOM? Learn how the "Word of Wisdom" prompted Dr. Christopher toward a higher way of healthy living. $1.75

DR. CHRISTOPHER'S NATURAL HEALING NEWSLETTERS Over six volumes of back issues that cover subjects ranging from distilled water to dandelions and the nervous system to nursing. 12 issues per volume. $2.75 each issue or $25.00 per volume.

A HEALTHIER YOU AUDIO NEWSLETTER Continuing series of newsletters in an audio cassette format. Listen to learn the current issues and research in the field of herbs and natural healing from David Christopher, M.H. -host of the weekly radio program "A Healthier You" now in its fifth year. One year subscription (12 issues) for $29.00

Available from: CHRISTOPHER PUBLICATIONS
P.O. Box 412 Springville, Utah 84663
or call toll free 1-800-372-8255

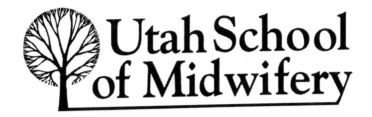

Utah School of Midwifery

The Utah School of Midwifery (USofM) was founded in 1980. The principal objective of the school is to provide education and training in the art and science of traditional, Christian midwifery. USofM offers pertinent midwifery curriculum. Today, midwifery students get their training mainly through apprenticing with experienced midwives. Understandably, many of these trainers do not have sufficient time to develop a curriculum for their trainees due to professional demands, family obligations, etc. Nor do many of them possess the pedagogical expertise to do so. The USofM provides such trainers and trainees with affordable correspondence training packages.

There are real benefits to midwifery training through correspondence. Such courses enable the trainees to pursue their education at their own pace and without having to leave family, friends, and employment. Trainees can locate midwives in their own area to apprentice with. A midwife is more likely to take on a trainee who has already completed some courses in midwifery and has a good understanding of the birth process and the role of an apprentice.

The USofM is associated and shares offices with The School of Natural Healing which was founded by Dr. John R. Christopher, N.D., M.H. and has been continually training Herbalists and natural healers longer than any other school in the United States.

The USofM courses are excellent for people interested in holistic health and self sufficiency. Students do not have to be aspiring midwives.

Curriculum Overview

The curriculum is divided into three areas of study: Birth Attendant, Labor and Delivery, and Prenatal and Postnatal Care. Students are free to pursue these areas of study in whatever order they want. However, USofM recommends that the students take the Birth Attendant courses first, since these courses present many of the basic midwifery concepts and terminology that are discussed in greater detail and depth in the other areas of study.

UTAH SCHOOL OF MIDWIFERY
Birth Attendant Home Study Courses

LS100 Introduction to Anatomy-Body Systems, 5 cr.

Course Overview: This course covers basic identification and functions of the various body systems--skin, skeletal, muscular, nervous, endocrine, circulatory, respiratory, digestive, urinary, and reproductive. Some of the material covers how pregnancy affects body systems.

Text:
1. Memmler & Wood, *The Human Body in Health and Disease,*

PHYS120 Body Works--Reflexology, 4 cr.

Course Overview: This course covers basic reflexology skills and specifically foot reflexology skills. Reflex points for the entire foot plus some reflex points on other parts of the body are covered. Reflex points for the body systems and specific disorders are also covered. Particular attention is given to pain relief and body work during labor. Principles of applied lymphology are explained. Students give 30 foot reflexology treatments and teach a class on reflexology.

Text:
1. Kunz/Kunz, *The Complete Guide to Foot Reflexology (Revised).*

HH130 Holistic Health, 4 cr.

Course Overview: This course covers health properties of various herbs. Information is given about herbal combinations for female disorders, pregnancy, and childbirth. Basic principles of holistic health, nutrition helps, and hydrotherapy techniques are covered. Students outline and teach a class on nutrition.

Texts:
1. John R. Christopher, *Herbal Home Health Care*
2. Thrash/Thrash, *Home Remedies*
3. Keith/Gordon, *The How To Herb Book*
4. Harvey and Marilyn Diamond, *Fit for Life*
5. Ann Wigmore, *The Wheatgrass Book*

HH131 Herb Identification and Preparations, 3 cr.

Course Overview: The material discusses plants and their parts, properties, and family names. Information is given to help students identify common herbs. Instructions are given for making different types of herbal preparations. The chemistry and action of herbs are delineated. Herbs used for specific body systems are identified.

Texts:
1. Max G. Barlow, *From The Shepherd's Purse*
2. Steven Foster, *Herbal Renaissance*

MDW140 Introduction to Midwifery, 4 cr.

Course Overview: The material discusses midwifery trainee/trainer relationship, labor coaching, taking vitals, charting, pelvimetry, fetal position, emergency childbirth, obstetrical drugs, setting up instruments and equipment, assessing post partum fundal height, placenta examination, clean up, birth certificates, birth statistics, and other basic skills of a birth attendant. Students outline and teach a class on labor coaching. The emphasis of this course is to prepare the student to be an apprentice midwife.

Texts:
1. Carolyn Steiger, *Becoming a Midwife*
2. Ina May Gaskin, *Spiritual Midwifery*
3. Elizabeth Davis, *Heart and Hands*
4. Stewart, Ph.D., *The Five Standards of Safe Childbearing*
5. Mendelsohn, *Confessions of a Medical Heretic*

Advanced Home Study Courses Include:

Prenatal and Postnatal Care

Medical Terminology, Genetics, Introduction to Iridology, Prenatal and Postnatal Care, Diagnostic Tests, and Pediatrics

Labor and Delivery

Anatomy and Physiology of Obstetrics, Body Work--Massage, Herbology, Labor and Delivery, Labor and Delivery Complications, and Traditional Midwifery

Students work on an individual course by going through the study guide, reading the text/s, completing the assignments, and then sending copies of their completed course work to USofM. The school examines the materials and returns it to the student. At the same time, USofM sends a test to measure the student's mastery of the subject to a proctor. The proctor administers the test to the student and then mails it back to USofM. Upon receiving the completed test, USofM grades the test, assigns a grade for the course, and then sends a transcript to the student that show the credits and grades for the course.

For more information write to: Utah School of Midwifery
Post Office Box 412
Springville, Utah 84663
or call 1-800-372-8255

NOTES

NOTES

NOTES